MW01601898

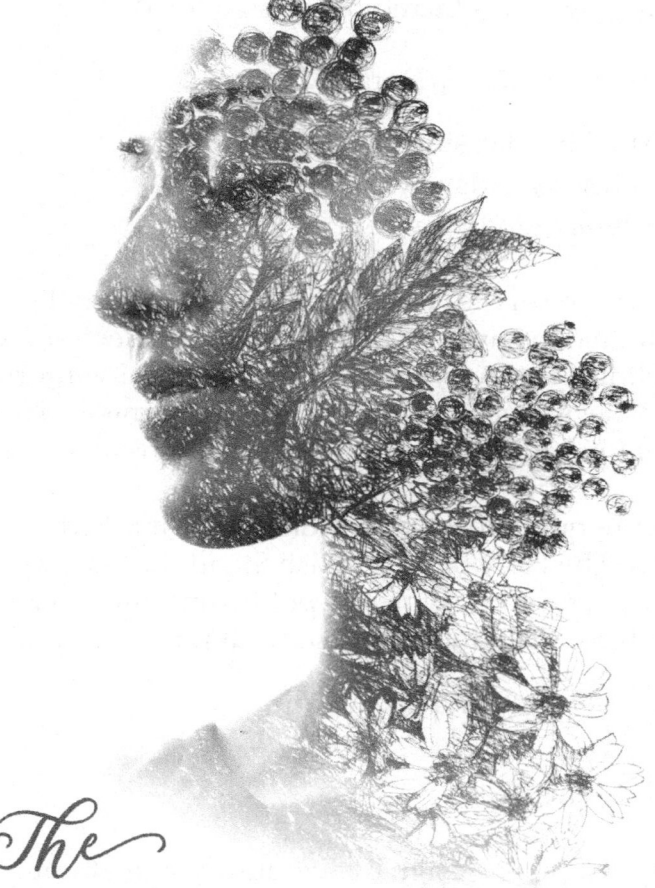

The
BLESSINGS *of* MAIDENHOOD
MATERNITY *&* MENOPAUSE

Celebrating God's Incredible Design for Women

DORAN RICHARDS

The Blessings of Maidenhood, Maternity & Menopause
Celebrating God's Incredible Design for Women

Published by: Blessing God's Way
www.blessinggodsway.com
info@blessinggodsway.com

ISBN: 9798645527211

First Edition: 2020

Cover and Book Design by Exodus Design Studio.

Printed in the United States of America

Dedication

Words that are worthy and holy don't come easy. The words written here, in this book, are for the encouragement, edification and inspiration of all women everywhere. It comes to you with a cost and sacrifice. I want to extend my uttermost, deep, heartfelt thanks and gratitude to my family for allowing me to walk out my calling and gifting; uplifting me along the way. I also want to thank all the women who have contributed to poems, songs, resources, and thoughts put in these pages. It truly takes a tribe, a family, to see something like this to fruition. May what is written here be a blessing to you and many more in the generations to come.

Table of Contents

I

An Introduction

I was *compelled* to write this book. I am sure you have heard that before, but this was something I felt I was called to do, for whatever reason. Only He knows.

I have worked seriously in the birthing realm for about 10 years. It started out with the home birth of my third child, Isaac. Before he was conceived, we had tried and tried to get pregnant. One day, my friend asked me to attend a midwifery conference that teaches about birth. I was a little skeptical but agreed nonetheless. This conference greatly altered my life. Patti Barnes, a midwife serving women in North Carolina, had come to share her wisdom with moms and young ladies interested in birth. She taught the women that having a baby is a normal life process, that their body is designed to give birth, and that it is not something to be feared. What an enlightening revelation! I remember asking her, "Patti, what would you tell your clients if they were `trying' to have a baby?" She replied by asking me if my husband drank coffee. I said, "Yes, and lots of it!" She then replied in her soft, sweet voice, "Well, I would tell him to stop. That can alter the sperm count and activity." So, I went home and reluctantly shared this news with my husband. Amazingly, he was open to cutting down but not quitting altogether. The next month we were pregnant!

Life was very different for me from then on. I went to a doctor's office that offered midwifery care. I knew that my body was made to birth. I knew that God designed the whole process and that I could trust Him. I knew that I didn't need all the tests and procedures that were pushed on me as a patient in my previous two hospital birth pregnancies. I knew that the word patient was the wrong word to use for what I was: I was a client, not a patient. Patient means you are sick. I was not sick, in fact, quite the opposite! The midwife, smiling and feeling sorry that she could not be of further help to me, said that I needed to have a home birth. Wow, the midwife was sending me home! That was such a strange sensation and a surreal situation. I quickly told her I didn't know of any midwives in my area that delivered at home. She said she would help me find someone because the office she worked at could not provide me with a normal and non-invasive birth experience, which is what I desired. This is where faith stepped in.

We trusted that God would provide for our needs. We trusted God that He would reveal to us His will for this birth. We prayed for those things because of our past two hospital experiences, which were less than desirable, and we prayed that God would protect us and guide us in this decision-making process. To top it all off, I was about 7 months along in the pregnancy.

That week, the midwife from the doctor's office called. She informed us that there was a midwife doing births in my area. She gave me her contact information, and we called right away. To our surprise, this midwife was able to come to our home and meet with us. She was willing to work with us, based on what we told her on the phone about our situation. What a blessing and an answer to prayer!

The midwife who came, Zan Ruby, was the sweetest lady you could ever possibly meet. As she entered our home, she sat on the floor and looked us in the eyes. She said she would be honored to help us and that she would love to attend our first homebirth. This was the confidence we were looking for. We were pleased beyond measure and so grateful for God's provision in bringing this midwife into our lives. My story is not a rare one, something I later found out as a midwife myself.

We had a beautiful baby boy at home that April. The birth was so normal that it seemed unreal. It was not a medicated birth, it was not rushed, and it didn't include any unnecessary interventions. I was able to allow my body to do the work it was made to do, naturally.

That is the beginning of how I got involved in the birthing realm. After that, I became active in my state, attempting to obtain licensure for the Certified Professional Midwives. I wanted to see all midwives able to attend births, whether at home, in the hospital, or at the birth center. Because midwifery care is different than the medical model that most women are familiar with, I set out to teach the midwifery model to all I knew, knowing that in most cases (especially in low-risk) it is a better way to birth. If you want more information on why midwifery care is as safe—if not safer—than the medical model, check out the Citizens for Midwifery website at www.cfmidwifery.org, where you can obtain fact sheets and various tools for teaching the midwifery model of care.

From there, I was surrounded by women and birth and started attending births with midwives to help them however I could. It was not in an official way, and not as an apprentice or student of midwifery, but solely to serve and help however I could. In this time of assisting, I learned a lot of new concepts and ideas that often surround birth. I learned that most people see that birth is spiritual as well as physical. I learned that women are fearful today and having children is not a top priority because they see it as a burden, illness, or inconvenience. I learned that women could feel alone and without support during this important time in their lives. This was all so disheartening to me. It was devastating to me, as a believer, to see something God calls blessed, rewarding, and a gift (children and pregnancy) turned into what it is today. This was not just outside the church universal, but inside it as well. Even we, as Christians, do not have a positive outlook on pregnancy and childbirth. Of course, there are always exceptions to the rule, but the overall experience of women during pregnancy and childbirth was concerning to me as a person, a developing midwife, and as a Christian.

I was invited one day to a *blessingway* ceremony for a friend who had worked on midwifery advocacy with me. I agreed to go, fascinated at the thought of a different kind of baby shower that honored the mother, and was mother-centered. This ceremony was eye-opening to me and a learning experience I will never forget. I remember there were a lot of women gathered, and they all offered such sweet gifts from their heart to the mother-to-be, encouraging her and uplifting her for the transition ahead. The amazing and most shameful thing that stood out in my mind was that no one gave credit where credit was due for the design and sustaining abilities of the pregnancy. God was not credited as the Creator of pregnancy, birth, and the mother's ability to carry a child. It was not even mentioned that it was by God alone that her womb was opened and she was pregnant. Oh, how sad this was to me.

Weeks after this ceremony, God spoke to me, and He spoke loudly for me to hear. I was to create a gathering that was God-honoring, God-glorifying, and God-centered. A gathering that brought women together to see God's work, to hear His word, to sing songs of praise; all components were to point the mother-to-be to God, and His design for pregnancy. How His grace is sufficient, His love is enduring, His provision is enough, and His grace is overflowing. Women in their last month of pregnancy need to hear these things. They need to taste and see that He is God and He is good.

Pregnancy is such a vulnerable time for women, and they are

more susceptible to the wiles of the devil. With hormonal changes taking place on a grand scale, it is harder to maintain a sense of balance and clarity. I wanted to create a gathering that pointed women to God as well as create a time of peace and fellowship. This would be done through singing, pampering, and reading the word, as well as offering prayer.

Serving one another is hard to do in our fast-paced lives. The task gets more and more cumbersome as we live our own lives and have so many things on our plate. Yet we are commanded to love one another, serve one another, and to lift one another up in times of need. Pregnancy is a time of need, and a God-centered Celebration of Pregnancy can provide a healthy perspective, support, and a feeling of love in a women's life when she needs it the most.

Blessing God's Way was then created as a Celebration of Pregnancy. It was created for women to replace the traditional, material-based baby showers, and for them to have a tool to serve one another. God's name has been taken out of the childbearing realm in our culture, especially in the secular world. I desire, with God's help, to bring His name back to the center of pregnancy and childbirth, where it should be. Why should it be? Because pregnancy and childbirth are blessings to us—God's way.

I want women to see that pregnancy and childbirth are a blessed gift from our Lord, and you can help. Pregnancy is a blessing, not a curse, and we need to realize and know that He is our Provider who offers us strength and grace when it is needed. Above all else, He is the One to receive the glory, honor, and praise for such a gift.

How does all of this relate to our other cycles? Well, let me explain a little further how Blessing God's Way emerged from an organization celebrating maternity to one that included maidenhood and menopause as well.

I taught at pregnancy-related conferences on topics such as erasing a spirit of fear, taking responsibility for your birth, trusting the birth process as God designed it, as well as the wonderful opportunity we have as sisters in Christ to serve one another. Women would come to me and comment on how the concepts I was teaching really applied to maidenhood and menopause, as well as maternity. It was an "aha" moment for me. Yes, I realized they were right; it certainly did apply to all three cycles in women's lives. All three cycles are often looked upon with disgust and discomfort. Women believe the lies of the culture around them that say those times are a curse, an illness, or that they are burdensome and less than desirable seasons of womanhood. How sad this is.

It doesn't have to be this way. God is not being honored with this mindset. His name has been taken out of these seasons (cycles), and that is not how it ought to be. We need to invite the Holy Spirit back into these seasons. Focus on the beauty of them. The revelation of God's grace. His mercy and glory for us as women. He designed our bodies to work so intricately and beautifully. We are truly fearfully and wonderfully made.

Let us go forth and teach the coming generations God's amazing design for our bodies, how they work, and how perfect His design is. Let us start here. By reading this book, you are taking the first step in this process of changing the tide of our current worldview. This can definitely have an impact inside the church. But consider the impact it could have on the church universal. It all begins individually, then moving through our churches and communities, it can spread and trickle onward and beyond to more than we could ever imagine. We need to commit to make a change and teach our daughters and sons the true design and concept of our cycles. We need to educate, support, and encourage them so they too can reap the blessings ten-fold.

Blessing God's Way Vision

We can change our culture's view if we work together. Let us point our sisters to our God, who alone is worthy, wise, and awesome. Come, join us in our efforts to spread this message.

There are many contributors to the deception surrounding women's beautifully designed bodies. Different cultures and belief systems carry myths and folklore that scare and oppress women into helplessness and even ignorance. Often, in the family unit, where we are supposed to be nurtured and protected, many women receive the wrong messages about their bodies and their purpose. This negativity grows as girls mature, and they find they are ill-equipped or afraid to teach the truth to their own daughters.

As some women struggle to regain some of their God-given heritage, there is little help to be found in the educational field. In the church, families are instructed in the ways of righteousness, but there is little to no discussion of the female body and its design. This leaves many women to turn to the culture and the media for answers about their life stages.

From a young girl's coming of age to her body's wonderful design in childbirth to the blessed mentoring stages of menopause, a woman needs to have accurate and truthful information. The time has come for us to step into the gap and equip women with the wonderful truths of God's word, which will then lead them to discover the beautiful symbolism in the design of their bodies! By learning about womanhood through scripture, women will be enabled to become mentors for the next generation.

Blessing God's Way seeks to provide communities with the tools to proclaim the amazing message of God's wondrous creation of the human body. We seek to be an international, non-denominational standard for implementing resources on the three branches of womanhood: Maidenhood, Maternity, and Menopause. Our hope is to see our culture recognize the importance of proclaiming God as the creator of women's cycles and educating women on His design.

Because of how far from God's design our culture has defined our phases of womanhood, creating a spirit of negativity and a feeling of doom, we are going to redefine these phases of womanhood in light of God's glorious design for us as women.

Maidenhood is defined as a time of blessing as girls mature into womanhood, and their bodies change physically, emotionally, and spiritually. It is also a time of discovery, where they learn how our Creator wonderfully and fearfully made them.

Maternity is defined as a time of blessing where women recognize how the Creator designed their bodies to experience pregnancy, labor, and postpartum. We desire for them to realize that it is a normal life process that is not just physical, but also a holistic event that encompasses all of our whole being, mind, body, and spirit.

Menopause is defined as a time of blessing as women embrace rest, renewal, and restoration through the ceasing of their monthly cycle. It is an acknowledgment of the Creator's plan for their bodies to come full circle, and a time to focus on maintaining health and contentment.

To Be A Blessing God's Way

by Michele Wheaton

Come now, Spirit, reveal your truth
Of woman, her legacy, design, and worth
For what, Creator, declares your glory?
From rib-to-woman tells your story.

Not lust of flesh, nor pride of life,
Vainglory, sensuality, nor strife;
Not dread, anxiety, fear or pain
Not shunned, confused, oppressed, or shamed.
But woman, I've made you to be
A testimony of love, of Me.

Maiden flower, blossoms wide
Child and woman awkwardly collide
Crimson red by cycle flows.
Draw near to Me, pour out your woes;
Hear my voice, be virtuous today
Exalt me and be,
A blessing God's way.

Mother, stretch your faith and trust
In I, your Lord- my grace is enough.
Sit at my feet, and sup with me;
Life grows within you, a miracle you'll see.
Women to mother, come alongside,
Labor, pray, and fortify.

Oh, life! How fearfully and wonderfully made!
For second birth, my Son, he paid.
On Christ's behalf, behold a babe!
Now to your breast, may this child lay.

Trust me and be,
A blessing God's way.
O woman, ripened now with years,
Who cycled, birthed and loved with tears,
Tarried on through harvest, stretched forth your hand,
Served others faithfully, by His command.
Far wiser, more beautiful, refined, and true,
God's great commission extends to you.

Will you surrender, commit to be,
My daughter, obedient, and teach others of me?
Adorned with good works, beautified, purified,
Holy as I am, mentoring life;
Lift high my name, and you will see
Your body, your purpose, I've created for me
To glorify my name, draw near the lost
By blood to blood, a sobering cost.

Christ, take my heart, to you I give
Prayerfully, on knee, I pledge to live
Speak now, Spirit, what can I do today?
To pass on the legacy
Of Blessing God's Way?

II

Cycle Worldview

"Boy, you have your hands full!"

"What number is that for you? Wow!"

"Have you heard of that new pill that takes away your period, so you don't have to endure it anymore?"

"Are you ready to have your uterus taken out? I sure am!"

What kind of comments do you hear surrounding the cycle you happen to be in? There are all kinds of negative thoughts, usually made without the true knowledge of that particular cycle. There are so many misconceptions and myths surrounding all phases of women's natural life cycle. History says our menstruation is a curse, pregnancy an illness to fix, and menopause the end of our life as we know it. Kind of dismal, isn't it? There isn't much hope for us ladies in that statement. We might as well throw in the towel and call it done.

Consider this comment from **Menstrual Musings** on the Glad Rags company website for cloth pads:

> *"The menstrual cycle is a healthy and natural process. However, in our culture we have been led to believe it is a messy inconvenience to be kept secret, or worse, a*

repugnant disease-like condition. We encourage you to examine your beliefs about menstruation carefully. Any embarrassment or shame you may feel could be the result of culturally inspired negative conditioning. How we perceive and interpret the feelings that accompany our cycles can have a dramatic effect on our health. Imagine the self-fulfilling destiny of the girl who hears, "Now you've got the curse, get ready for cramps, and a bloody mess."

The reason we want to counter this mindset is that it goes beyond our first cycle; it bleeds (excuse the pun) into the other cycles we will experience as well. It mainly affects our cycles of maternity and menopause. We have a chance to practice a good attitude, not a poor one. It starts at the beginning, and it can be taught to your daughters as early as they can retain and understand the information.

For maternity, this comment from a doula organization hits home as far as our mindset for pregnancy and maternity today:

"The fact is, society has become so anti-child that people are actually pressured into `excusing' their children as toys or hobbies. Women rave about their `marvelous experience' of childbirth more than they do about the child himself or herself. Motherhood must become chic in order to be justified. All those cute T-shirts for pregnant women with `Mommy' stenciled on them, all those cute coordinated quilts for baby's room, are not proof that our culture overflows with love for children. They prove, rather that children have been resurrected as pets. - Mary Pride, **The Way Home, Beyond Feminism - Back to Reality**

This is what the current worldview would have us believe:

- Pregnancy is an illness.
- Pregnancy is a medical event to be managed.
- Pregnancy is a disaster waiting to happen.
- Pregnancy is a burden, curse, hardship, and financial strain.

But, biblically, we should really see maternity this way:

- Pregnancy is a reward and a gift from our Father in heaven.
- Pregnancy is an honor and privilege.
- Pregnancy should be a time of joy and celebration.
- Pregnancy is an extension of His kingdom here on earth.

God warns us about falling into the trap of walking with the world and not being separate and holy, as He is holy.

> *"Do not be conformed to this world, but be transformed by the renewal of your mind, that by testing you may discern what is the will of God, what is good and acceptable and perfect."* Romans 12:2

My heart aches when I see the faces of women who are pregnant. It is like their whole life is just hanging by a thread. Women look tired, alone, disinterested , and apathetic. Women do not want to educate themselves on this wonderful cycle because they are afraid or discouraged. God has been so gracious to us as women. His design is perfect. We are, for certain, fearfully and wonderfully made. If only we could only teach this to our next generation by changing the tide of our beliefs on pregnancy, we might see more women embracing their God-given cycle instead of the concept of "running away" from it that is so rampant in our culture.

In our last cycle, menopause, women are again led through a false worldview on how their cycle should be perceived. Instead of looking at our bodily changes in a positive light, we navigate towards the negative images, becoming discouraged by the modern perception of natural aging.

We don't realize how prevalent the negativity becomes until we really begin to think about how destructively it has affected our culture. I am not only speaking of the secular culture, but rather the Christian community as well, and how it has lost it's vision. The vision that is missing is that God created these cycles, and that they have spiritual, physical, and emotional implications that can either lead us to or away from Christ. This book will address some of the spiritual, physical, and emotional aspects of our cycles and how we can be supportive and encouraging to our sisters within the church universal. Let us help each other envision how our cycles are blessings to us, God's way (you will see me repeat this often, but repetition is always a great tool in remembering a good concept)!

> *"Do you not know that your bodies are members of Christ?"* I Corinthians 6:15

> *"Look carefully then how you walk, not as unwise but as wise, making the best use of the time, because the days are evil. Therefore do not be foolish, but understand what the will of the Lord is."* Ephesians 5:15-17

III

Owning Our Cycles

*"The man who complains about the way the ball bounces
is likely to be the one who dropped it."*
Lou Holtz, Hall of Fame football coach

We need to take responsibility for our bodies and our cycles. We need to research and know how they work and why they work this way. What are the ramifications of this design, and how does it affect me? How can I teach a positive aspect of this design to my daughters? We need to see the importance of using these seasons as opportunities to teach about God's goodness, mercy, and faithfulness to us as women. There are so many significant aspects of each cycle, and I think you will be truly amazed to learn about them. The result of the learning process is "owning it," and also understanding that we are not to be ignorant about how God has designed our bodies. He tells us to get wisdom and to understand. The scriptures are full of exhortations to get knowledge and wisdom. Why would our cycles and how they work be any different? God can be revealed in all things, even in our cycles. This is truly amazing!

"Your doctor has NOT been trained to take care of healthy women. He has been trained to take care of sick people. Your pregnancy is not a disease or a sickness. Your doctor will treat your pregnancy [and your other cycles, for that matter] as if it is a disease to be managed. But you have hit the nail on the head when you say that it's EASIER to let the doctor handle everything. Most people do not want to be bothered with learning the things that are necessary to be healthy. It's not as hard as you might think. You don't have to go to school or get a degree. The information you need in order to have a healthy birth {or to be able to embrace the cycle God has you in} is available to everyone, and you don't have to be a doctor to understand it. Most people simply don't want to be bothered or don't want the responsibility. That is why doctors get sued for malpractice—people want someone else to be responsible if something goes wrong."

- The Center for Unhindered Living, ***Autonomous Pregnancy and Birth*** [my emphasis added in brackets]

This quote reveals a sad example of how women fail to take responsibility. The furthest they go is making an appointment with someone who is trained in fixing illnesses instead of searching the Bible for answers and seeking Godly women's advice for how to embrace and walk through that particular cycle. Don't get me wrong, medical professionals are blessings for when we need them, for medical emergencies or illnesses that require their expertise, but our cycles as a whole are not such events.

For our young ladies who are getting ready to embark on their first cycle of menses, they need good resources to see this as a positive experience. One of the first places they learn from is their mothers. They should be taught that God created it from the beginning and that He created it for our good, for a cleansing, for a renewing, which is beautiful and wonderful!

Many young ladies are being left to understand menstruation on their own, surrounded by the negative secular world, and they can't be expected to always view it in a positive light. All healthy women experience menstruation for most of their lives. Yet it is a topic cloaked in secrecy, taboo, and negativity; few women see the merits of menstruation. Many people believe that menstruation is dirty and disgusting. How is it possible that a major part of the experience of being a woman is viewed with such disdain and denial? Negative views of menstruation are common, and their sources and implications deserve increased consideration.

For women entering menopause, they also don't have many resources available to them. Secular resources abound, but they don't point to God, who created menopause. They really give credit to everyone but God. God created all our cycles for a purpose. Getting information on our cycle and how it applies to us as Christians will help us gain confidence. It will help us not to have fear surrounding it, and it will also enable us to actually celebrate the cycle in a wholesome way, not in a secular, humanistic, and feministic way. We will talk more about celebrating each cycle later in this book.

So how do we take responsibility and own our cycles in a Godly way? First of all, we read the scriptures, asking God to reveal to us the seasons in our lives and how what He has created is good. We should seek out individuals who can encourage and support us through the cycles. We can write more pamphlets and articles and books from a Christian point of view if we are gifted in this area. All of our lives have spiritual implications.

> *"There is a ton of misinformation out there.so just make sure you do the research, so you don't fall into the trap that so many parents in our culture have fallen into blindly following the cultural trends. These trends are often unhealthy for families and can be especially detrimental to children, and some common beliefs are just simply false information! Only you can decide what is*

right for you and your family. So in order to make an informed decision, you have to do the research."

- Tina Smith, www.fresnofamily.com

It is your responsibility. You have to be discerning when obtaining information on any of the three phases; there are false facts surrounding them all. We are all guilty of falling into the trap set by the culture of being ignorant and ill-informed. What do we do about it? We repent and go and sin no more!

We need to take responsibility for our own health and outcomes. This means not transferring our responsibility to others through a lack of knowledge. The word ignorance has a negative connotation, but it simply means a lack of knowledge on a particular subject. Let us ask God to forgive us for our ignorance and our lack of understanding and to help us do better about obtaining the understanding and wisdom concerning His design for us.

> *"See to it that no one takes you captive by philosophy and empty deceit, according to human tradition, according to the elemental spirits of the world, and not according to Christ."* Colossians 2:8

When we obtain knowledge, however, we have to make sure not to shove it down someone else's throat. We all have different walks with God and we are all at different stages and maturity levels. Where I may be in my understanding is not where you might be in yours. Let us walk in grace, encouraging one another to get knowledge. Let us aspire to gain understanding and wisdom about our cycle and phases of womanhood with a spirit of love, uplifting, and mentoring in our hearts in a Godly manner. That is what will speak mountains to our friends and family as well as the culture around us.

Have you thought about how the lack of knowledge and education has become so rampant? How has education on our cycle, within the church universal, been eliminated from our teachings within our homes and churches? One main reason that our cycles are not being taught from a biblical perspective is that most of our leadership in the churches is, understandably, male. Men in that position often do not realize the need to teach on the cycles, believing them to be a topic better handled by the medical community, or even just passed from mothers to daughters in the home. This is detrimental to our beliefs on these cycles. They do have spiritual aspects as well as physical and emotional.

> *"It's time for the Church to wake up and reclaim birth {and our other phases of womanhood} as the spiritual blessing God intended. It's also time to reintegrate faith, Biblical truths, and Titus 2 modeling back into birthing [and our other phases as women]. When we do, we will begin not only to see healthier birth outcomes, but reclamation of the family by providing them with a happier and healthier foundation."*

- Kathy Rateliff, Certified Christian Doula, Christian Childbirth Educator, and Cord Blood Educator, [emphasis added.]

God's name has been taken out of these realms in our lives. He has been forgotten, forsaken, and disregarded in each of our phases of life. We can change this and rebuild communities in order for them to see the importance of the cycles. But not so much that we lift them up and worship them. No, that would be sinful. We do not worship the cycle but the One who created the cycle. He demands the glory and says so in His word:

> *"Not to us, O Lord, not to us, but to your name give glory, for the sake of your steadfast love and your faithfulness!"*
> Psalm 115:1

And again:

> *"Declare his glory among the nations, his marvelous works among all the peoples!"* Psalm 96:3

He wants us to give Him glory for all things, and our cycles should not be excluded from this command. He wants the glory for how we are so fearfully and wonderfully made (Psalm 139:13-16). He wants us to be lights that so shine before men that we may glorify our Father in heaven (Matthew 5:16). We can be shining lights during our cycles, giving our secular world a proper view and insight into what our cycles are and why they were created for our good. Let our glow in pregnancy be that of the Holy Spirit, revealing His design to the nations!

Owning our cycle means that we realize all of this. That God created us and He created us with a purpose. We have a responsibility to search out the matter of our cycle, whichever one we are in at the time, and teach it from a Godly perspective to the next generation. The culture has a very poor view of our natural cycles right now, but we as Christians can change that, one family at a time. Now is the time to make that change. The rebuilding has to begin with us: Christian women who want to recognize and glorify God in all things.

There are many tools for obtaining knowledge on our cycles:

- The Bible
- Books
- DVDs
- Support groups
- Fact sheets (it is so easy to "google" information)
- Sharing positive stories

To start change, we need to be active and do something about it. Blessing God's Way ministry is a tool for just this type of action. Please use it and take advantage of it, as a tool to teach women the beauty of God's design. All three cycles are truly blessings to us, God's way!

IV

Fearful Spirits

One of the main reasons we have such a hard time embracing our God-given cycles is because of the "f" word—FEAR! Instead of trusting the process, we fear it. We will talk about the trusting process in the next chapter. For now, let's explore what it means to erase a spirit of fear surrounding our cycles.

First of all, God tells us not to have a spirit of fear for anything except a fear of Him. We cannot begin to truly celebrate our design as women until we learn how to erase a spirit of fear and to trust the process of our cycles.

> *"…for God gave us a spirit not of fear but of power and love and self-control."* II Timothy 1:7

For maidenhood, young girls have trepidation about their first arriving cycle. They may be anxious because they are not sure what it entails. Maternity is another area where fear grows and expands rapidly. In menopause, women refuse to understand fully what their body is about to go through, because of the fear that surrounds it as well. Why is this? It is because of the culture we live in, no doubt.

In most instances, this is a spirit of fear. It is a fear of the unknown. As humans, we want to control and know everything.

That is what makes us comfortable and safe. Well-seasoned Christians will tell you this is not so, that it is not walking in faith, but truly by sight. We need to walk in faith, trusting, and knowing that God has ordained these cycles and that they are in His hands. They always have been and always will be. His grace is sufficient, even for menses, maternity, and menopause. Young girls may be fearful because of stories they hear at school or church. They may be made fun of, or simply be afraid everyone will know when they are having their menstruation. Pregnant women often fear birth, pain, and the work of raising children. Menopausal women are scared of the process of their cycle ceasing or waning, and hormones controlling their lives as well as driving them crazy. We need support. We need our fellow Christian sisters pointing us to God, who alone is wise and merciful.

One definition of fear is an anxious concern. This describes what women in all three cycles experience to some degree. Having a spirit of fear does not please God, but it does please Satan. We do not want to hand him our weakness to prey upon and use against us. This is a very real problem in today's society concerning our cycles.

We have many different areas that are touched and affected by this. Our family is influenced by how we perceive our cycles. Our daughters and sons will learn from us, whether or not it is a blessing or a curse. It is important to have positive reactions and to handle these cycles well. We should bless God and praise Him for our cycle, not complain and murmur against our loving God.

Our community is touched in one way or another by how we embrace our cycles. When you are in the grocery store, and you experience a hot flash or someone's cruel look for how many children you happen to be toting along, what will you do? Will you greet people around you with a smile and love, or will you have a depressed and sad countenance about you? You can either shine for God or look fearful of the situation you are in.

There is a process to having a spirit of fear. Kelly Townsend, in her book, *Christ Centered Childbirth* explains that fear:

- Begins in the thought realm;
- Moves to the emotional realm;
- Affects the physical realm;
- Attacks the volitional realm.

Try to understand how it begins with your thoughts. Taking your thoughts captive is essential. See how it moves to the emotional realm of that "uh-oh" feeling, where your stomach sinks, and you begin to feel sick. In the physical realm, your muscles will tighten, and you might become tense or have a headache. It ends in a place where you lack the ability to make correct choices for the situation you are in. You have lost the ability to think clearly. She is speaking about pregnancy and childbirth in her book, but it applies to the other cycles of life as well. It is amazing when you break it down to inspect each realm. I love this quote:

> *"Faith attracts the positive. Fear attracts the negative."*
> - Edwin Louis Cole, founder of the Christian
>   Men's Network

We should say this over and over again until the blessings that God intended are revealed to us, and we can take our thoughts captive. In turn, our fear does not keep us in bondage. Taking your thoughts captive takes time, energy, and practice. You will not have the ability to do so all of a sudden.

To be able to start practicing, you must begin with your thoughts, trusting in Him, and taking comfort in His assurance by faith. You have scriptures, good books, positive stories, generations of good outcomes, DVDs, and so much more in today's society to help you take your thoughts captive.

The main exercise in taking your thoughts captive is to pray, meditating on God's goodness and mercy. Seek His grace and stay seated at the foot of the cross to be able to see the right perspective. God tells us not to fear and to lay our burdens down. I love this quote:

> *"Rather than focusing on the goodness and strength of God, we focus on impending disasters, with God only coming in as an afterthought. It is easy to see that the discipline of developing a sound mind is something we all need to cultivate. A sound mind is a mind that can enjoy peace even in the midst of a great storm because it is anchored in what is really true."*

> - Elyse Fitzpatrick, *Overcoming Fear, Worry & Anxiety*

This is an excellent book, and I recommend that every woman read it sometime during her three cycles! We only see God as an afterthought, which is shameful. Focus is extremely important. Focus means "a concentrated effort or attention on a particular thing, an area of concern or responsibility, or the condition of seeing sharply and clearly." Can you relate this to being fearful of a cycle or season we are in? God tells us that a thousand may fall at our side, but it shall not come near us. He protects us and stays us.

> *"He who dwells in the shelter of the Most High will abide in the shadow of the Almighty."* Psalm 91:1

We need to focus on God's presence, His love, His beauty, and His everlasting covenant with His people, as well as His truth. His truth will set us free—free of fear! Philippians 4 lays out how we can take our thoughts captive. Go through these bullets and see how they truly can erase a spirit of fear and replace it with a spirit of trust and truth.

Philippians 4

- Obey God's command not to be anxious (verse 6)
- Call on the Lord in prayer (verse 6)
- Realize God's promise to keep your mind safe (verse 7)
- Meditate on God's Word and good things (verse 8)
- Learn and focus on Godly behavior (verse 9)
- Aim to help others, shifting your attention from yourself (verse 10)
- Learn to be content (verse 11)
- Rely on Christ's strength to help you (verse 13)
- Accept God's provision to meet your needs (verse 19)
- Realize that God's grace is with you (verse 23)

I would like to end this section with another quote by Elyse Fitzpatrick:

> *"As you face your fears—fears of suffering, fears of failure, fears of trouble and tribulation—you can know for certain that the God who loved you enough to send His son to die for you is still ruling the universe. If, in His loving plan, you have to bow before what appears to be a frowning providence, you can be sure that He's got your ultimate happiness at heart. He is working to free you from your worries—not by giving you freedom from trouble, but by arranging circumstances so that as you go through them you'll experience the truth that He is everything He says he is."*

- Elyse Fitzpatrick, **Overcoming Fear, Worry & Anxiety**

Now that is powerful. Maybe you could go back and read that excerpt again. I know I never tire of reading it!

V

Trusting God's Design

How can we trust the design that God has given us? We should trust it to be good, useful, needed, and productive. Our culture tells us all of the opposite things. Our culture, as we have already learned, calls maidenhood, maternity, and menopause burdens, sicknesses, and curses. It is almost inconceivable to trust Him because we are flooded with these lies constantly. Eventually, if we continue to heed our culture, we will believe the lies and myths. However, we are to be set apart and not conformed to this world. So how can we trust the processes of our cycles?

The number one problem with our trust is that it is not in God's design, but in the medical community. We often trust what they have to say about it without even questioning it.

You can see this in menstruation. We worry about starting late, starting too soon, excessive bleeding, pain, etc. Our first notion would be to take our daughters (or ourselves) to the doctor when any "complication" arises. Today, young girls are offered and prescribed pills to ease their pain and discomfort during their menstruation, and not only that, but something even more terrifying is happening. Young girls and women alike are given a certain type of pill to stop their period altogether! This mindset does not trust in God's design; instead, it is actively refusing to have faith in His care for your well-being. Our periods are given to us for a reason; they are used for cleansing and for a purification process. He created our bodies to clean themselves with blood. The powerful picture of blood, as a cleaning agent, is nothing new to Christians. If only we could teach this to our daughters before they are sold the lie that it is a nuisance and burden, how much more pleasing to God this would be.

Trusting the birth process is essential for a good birth outcome. I once listened to a midwife receive an award for her service in the community. As she was giving thanks and sharing a few words, she explained to her audience that over all the years that she had given care to women and families, she realized the one major lesson she had learned was to trust the process. I do not know if she was a Christian, but I would have said to trust *God's* process. He designed the body to do what it will do. He created most low-risk, healthy women to give birth without the aid of drugs and interventions.

Interventions are usually given because the process isn't trusted to continue on its own. Induction happens because, for the most part, the people involved do not trust the timing of God. There are always exceptions when those interventions and inductions are needed, but how often do we turn to them before turning to God and seeking His grace and wisdom in the process?

For menopause, women are sold lies from our culture that their uterus needs to be removed for them to live a healthy life. They believe that getting rid of that organ is the only answer to eliminating all the discomfort. This can sometimes be standard protocol. We should consider, however, that God gave us our organs for a reason. We really shouldn't be so quick to accept what advice we get from others in that respect without seeking out natural alternatives and support from our loving Christian sisters and church family. Pause and consider that trust is everything. It speaks mountains. It will give us the confidence to walk in God's will and to be those lights ourselves so that we will shine and glorify God in heaven. Take a look at how many scriptures refer to fully and wholly trusting in God.

Scriptures for TRUST

"Offer right sacrifices, and put your trust in the LORD." Psalm 4:5

"And those who know Your name will put their trust in You, for You, O LORD, have not forsaken those who seek You." Psalm 9:10

"Oh, guard my soul, and deliver me! Let me not be put to shame, for I take refuge in you." Psalm 25:20

"I hate those who pay regard to worthless idols, but I trust in the LORD." Psalm 31:6

"But I trust in You, O LORD; I say, `You are my God.'" Psalm 31:14

"For our heart is glad in Him, because we trust in His holy name." Psalm 33:21

"Trust in the LORD and do good; dwell in the land and befriend faithfulness." Psalm 37:3

"Commit your way to the LORD; trust in Him, and He will act." Psalm 37:5

"He put a new song in my mouth, a song of praise to our God. Many will see and fear, and put their trust in the LORD. Blessed is the man who makes the LORD his trust, who does not turn to the proud, to those who go astray after a lie!" Psalm 40:3-4

"For not in my bow do I trust, nor can my sword save me." Psalm 44:6

"But I am like a green olive tree in the house of God. I trust

in the steadfast love of God forever and ever." Psalm 52:8

"When I am afraid, I put my trust in You. In God, whose word I praise, in God I trust; I shall not be afraid. What can flesh do to me?" Psalm 56:3-4

"Trust in Him at all times, O people; pour out your heart before Him; God is a refuge for us. Put no trust in extortion; set no vain hopes on robbery; if riches increase, do not set your heart on them." Psalm 62:8, 10

"Because they did not believe in God and did not trust His saving power." Psalm 78:22

"Trust in the LORD with all your heart, and do not lean on your own understanding." Proverbs 3:5

"That your trust may be in the LORD, I have made them known to you today, even you." Proverbs 22:19 29

"Trust in the LORD forever, for the LORD GOD is an everlasting rock." Isaiah 26:4

"And again, `I will put my trust in Him.' And again, `Behold, I and the children God has given me.'" Hebrews 2:13

There are other avenues that we trust before God, not just the medical community. We trust the media (TV, radio, DVDs), our community, schools, Internet, and the generations of families who have gone before us. Trusting in God first is not the norm. It is a struggle and battle sometimes to hold on to trusting God first and foremost. Our intentions are good, but somehow we find ourselves in the same situation of traveling on the wide path and not the straight and narrow. I love how Mrs. Rochell explains this in her article, Developing the Capacity to Trust God:

"How then do we develop a greater trust in God, and put to rest our fears, doubts, and the `What if's' that emerge

when we attempt to give over more of our lives to divine will? It is one thing to want to have more faith in God, and it is quite another to live this kind of trust in a daily way. It is in the arena of our daily lives that we fully develop the capacity to trust God."

- Mashubi Rochell, Spiritual Counselor and Founder of World Blessings

This quote applies to our duty and calling of trusting in our cycle and the rest of our seasons. Trust is a beautiful attribute to have. We can continually cultivate this attribute and practice it in order to improve each day. We will not achieve perfection, but we can thank God we have this as a goal, and we can support and encourage one another to trust in Him!

VI

Numbers Are Prime

Numbers are important, especially to God. We can see this throughout the Bible, and we should try to comprehend why they are so important because it could be beneficial in understanding His plan. There are so many numbers and pictures about numbers that are represented in birth and other cycles. This section will take a look at some of them.

Let's start with the number 40. Forty weeks (the time of approximate gestation for pregnancy) is a number God uses over and over for transitions that bring about great change and blessings. The number 40 is often understood as the "number of probation or trial." For example: The Israelites wandered for 40 years (Deuteronomy 8:2-5); Moses was on the mount for 40 days (Exodus 24:18); 40 days were involved in the story of Jonah and Nineveh (Jonah 3:4); Jesus was tempted for 40 days (Matthew 4:2); and there were 40 days between Jesus' resurrection and ascension (Acts 1:3). He describes to us that these times are for testing our hearts and minds, and that, in the end, the "promised land" is oh, so sweet to behold, making it all worthwhile!

> *"The whole commandment that I command you today you shall be careful to do, that you may live and multiply, and go in and possess the land that the Lord swore to give to*

your fathers. And you shall remember the whole way that the Lord your God has led you these forty years in the wilderness, that he might humble you, testing you to know what was in your heart, whether you would keep his commandments or not. For the Lord your God is bringing you into a good land, a land of brooks of water, of fountains and springs, flowing out in the valleys and hills. And you shall eat and be full, and you shall bless the Lord your God for the good land he has given you."
Deuteronomy 8:1-10

On average, most women menstruate for about 40 years. There is that number again. Wow, God is good, isn't He? To give us such wonderful assurance that there is a new beginning after those 40 years of menstruation discomforts!

There are also visual pictures in the Bible that we can draw from in our life cycles. For example: the re-birth into the Kingdom of Heaven, or specifically, the process of being born again. When you are born again, it is with water, by being baptized. Water is extremely important; it is one of life's staples. It cleanses as well as nourishes us. In birth, water is used to cushion the baby through the process of being born in the canal. With the born again process, you are in darkness and brought into the light by the illumination of the Holy Spirit. The baby is in the womb (darkness) and goes through water (like the Red Sea or baptism), into the light of the world. Is water involved here by chance? Or to help us see God's goodness and mercy?

There is also the picture of Christ's blood being shed, once and for all, so that we may "enter in" and be born again. It is fascinating how blood is involved in all three of our cycles of maidenhood, maternity, and menopause.

In our first cycle, menstruation, we see that blood occurs monthly due to our bodies cleansing themselves for renewal and a fresh start. The blood is acting as a cleansing agent. We can see that the big picture of this is the knowledge and imagery of Christ's blood cleansing us from our sin. On a smaller scale, blood was shed to cover sins in the Old Testament; it was shed continuously so that God's chosen people may be cleansed and holy—"because He is holy." Girls need to know that their cycle is a beautiful agent God created to cleanse us and that, in and of itself, it is incredible!

In pregnancy, blood is part of the birthing process. It is cleansing; cleansing the uterus out of the placenta and bag of waters, and all the components of growing a baby inside your body. The body needs to go back to its normal state, and blood is a part of birth to do just that. Like our menstruation, maternity is normal; it is used as a blessing, not a curse. Teaching this will help all of us view pregnancy from a biblical perspective. God says, *"Your hands have made me and fashioned me, an intricate unity."* (Job 10:8) We are often fearful or unsure of each of these stages and what they entail, but God says, *"For God has not given us a spirit of fear."* (II Timothy 1:7) God declares that gaining knowledge is important so that we may obtain understanding and wisdom. *"Get wisdom! Get understanding! Wisdom is the principle thing; therefore, get wisdom."* (Proverbs 4:3) All of these scriptures apply to maidenhood, maternity and menopause.

In menopause, blood is ceasing or waning. There is a reason for that. Menopause is derived from the Greek words *mēn* (month) and *pausis* (pause/stop). God is giving you another aspect to life, another blessing, by taking that cleansing season and ending it. I believe God uses this season to give us a new beginning. It is a season to be grateful for because God has ordained this as a complete cycle that lasts for approximately 40 years. He is giving us a time of peace and a new, refreshed outlook on life. It is a "promised land" of sorts.

There is definitely suffering in our cycles. They can be uncomfortable and can require some extra support to stay

Christ-focused. There is pain and physical labor involved in getting to the new life from the old life, transitioning from being in the womb to the new life in the outside world.

Once I was at a birth, and the woman in labor was concentrating immensely on her pushing stage and was doing so well with taking her thoughts captive and staying focused on Christ. She said out loud in a cry of prayer, "Why is there suffering to get to the joy? Oh, why is there pain to get to the good side!" This was during the transition stage, right before the baby comes out and makes an appearance into this world. It is incredible that we can see this with Jesus' death on the cross. He suffered but eventually entered into the holiest of holies. And the Israelites went through so much toil, hardship, pain of hunger, and disbelief before they got to the Promised Land. It was encouraging to this woman for her to see that the pain and toil was a good sensation with a glorious ending—how beautiful!

I also marvel at how the baby, when born into the life outside the womb, takes a breath for the first time. It is a deep, life-filling breath. It is just like how we, as believers, are filled with the breath of the Holy Spirit when we are born again. We have a new life, and we ask for the breath of heaven to entangle us as we venture on this new journey. When babies take their first breath, it is incredible. It is a picture of our first breath in our new life as believers.

VII

The Lost Art of Serving

Being examples for Christ goes hand in hand with being a Christian and serving our LORD. Being pregnant does not mean that we are exempt from this duty, making ourselves not useful to serve our King. Quite the contrary; it is an opportunity to serve God, carrying a child for His good pleasure. We seem to think that this applies to raising children for God, but not actually carrying one in our wombs. Carrying a child for our LORD is an awesome way we can serve Him, and in doing so, we can be examples of the love of God. How can we keep this concept of "servanthood" to our LORD while we are pregnant? Ladies need encouragement, admonishing, and uplifting throughout the whole childbearing process, always reminding and pointing them to Christ, our King.

We are an example by looking to Christ and giving Him praise continually in our cycles. We often feel our cycles are burdensome because we are human, and we get overwhelmed. This is because we are not sufficient in and of ourselves. We must rely on the work of the Holy Spirit within us, sanctifying us daily to be more and more conformed to the image of Christ. Yes, even in our seasons of life through maidenhood, maternity, and menopause.

Our purpose on this earth is not to serve ourselves; it is to serve our Almighty God. If we are concentrating on our woes, giving in to fear, going about our daily lives with our agenda, we are bound to spiritual destruction. We might be neglecting our duties to carry out His agenda in our lives. What is God's agenda for your life? If we are seeking to do His will alone, there is no room for our own. Let us keep the truth of our service as children of God at the forefronts of our minds, teaching it to others by our example. Pregnancy is a golden opportunity to show this truth.

> *"Do you not know that your bodies are members of Christ?"* I Cor. 6:15

> *"Look carefully then how you walk, not as unwise but as wise, making the best use of the time, because the days are evil. Therefore do not be foolish, but understand what the will of God is."* Ephesians 5:15-17

I love how Paul Tripp in his book, **Instruments in the Redeemer's Hands**, states:

> *"God has placed His glory on us so that our lives and ministry would reveal Him on earth."*

This is so true even within all stages of our lives as women.

> *"...That those who live should no longer live for themselves but for Him who for their sake died and was raised."* II Cor. 5:15

Let us live for our God, for His glory, bringing all praise to Him for His good works. He has bestowed a child upon us, a glorious gift. Let our actions, as examples, shine brightly so that people see the brilliant glow of God on our faces!

> *"For if we live, we live to the LORD, and if we die, we die to the LORD."* Romans 14:8

God has given us many scriptures in the Bible pertaining to different aspects of celebrating our cycles. By being a host to women for a Celebration Gathering, or by serving one another in other ways during our cycles, we can begin to exhort, admonish, and encourage the women around us through them.

> *"As each has received a gift, use it to serve one another, as good stewards of God's varied grace: whoever speaks, as one who speaks oracles of God; whoever serves, as one who serves by the strength that God supplies — in order that in everything God may be glorified through Jesus Christ. To Him belong the glory and dominion forever and ever. Amen."* I Peter 4:10-11

How can we serve one another? How can we love one another? A Celebration Gathering gives us an opportunity to serve our fellow "sister in Christ" by setting aside a time to honor the LORD for His work in a loved one's life. Pampering the mother, daughter, aunt, or grandmother — and helping her to be spiritually fed by God's word for her transition — is essential in our role as friends and family.

How often do we wash each other's feet? How often do we humble ourselves in service toward others? We serve our families at home day by day. However, extending our love through service to others has become obsolete in our society with today's busy schedules. You can change this by offering a little of your time to serve others outside of your home through hosting a Celebration Gathering for someone you know. What an example of servanthood this would be to our young daughters and future generations!

We will talk more about celebrating in a moment, but for now, we need to know that gathering is a good thing, especially gathering around women to support and love them because it is so crucial for healthy relationships. We have an opportunity, as sisters in Christ, to meet and admonish one another throughout our cycles of life. Hospitality means treating guests with warmth and generosity. Celebration Gatherings offer a time that you can practice hospitality. Bringing fellow women and families into our homes gives us an opportunity to be an example of Christ and what He has done for us.

> *"Love one another with brotherly affection. Outdo one another in showing honor. Do not be slothful in zeal, be fervent in spirit, serve the LORD. Rejoice in hope, be patient in tribulation, be constant in prayer. Contribute to the needs of the saints and seek to show hospitality."* Romans 12:10-13

Did you know you could use so many of your wonderful Godly characteristics by hosting or attending a Celebration Gathering? Or by teaching a *Maidens by His Design* workshop in your community?

My call to you is to teach the women surrounding you— especially our daughters who are in the years between graduation from high school and marriage—that they can serve in a great capacity in their community. Oftentimes, young ladies find themselves idle during this season in their lives, yet if they only knew how needed they are in serving and supporting other young ladies and women during their cycles, they would be introduced to a whole new area of encouragement and nourishment.

My intention for writing this book is not only to celebrate these cycles by embracing them in a biblical way, but also to convert women's hearts for service to one another in these celebrations. The Holy Spirit changes our hearts and minds. He guides us, teaches us, and gives us understanding that we might be pleasing unto the LORD. I pray that you will see servanthood and hospitality in the proper light and that the Lord God Almighty would be glorified by any revelation you may receive by reading this book.

There are all kinds of scriptures that deal with "one anothers" and I think that would be a glorious way to end this chapter, listing them for your reading pleasure. They are, after all, how we are united in Him, and they give us instruction on how to serve another.

"One Another" Scriptures for Women

"Love one another with brotherly affection. Outdo one another in showing honor." Romans 12:9-11

"Rejoice with those who rejoice, weep with those who weep. Live in harmony with one another. Do not be haughty, but associate with the lowly. Never be wise in your own sight. Repay no one evil for evil, but give thought to do what is honorable in the sight of all." Romans 12:15-17

"Pay to all what is owed to them: taxes to whom taxes are owed, revenue to whom revenue is owed, respect to whom respect is owed, honor to whom honor is owed. Owe no one anything, except to love each other, for the one who loves another has fulfilled the law." Romans 13:7-9

"Therefore let us not pass judgment on one another any longer, but rather decide never to put a stumbling block or hindrance in the way of a brother." Romans 14:13

"Therefore welcome one another as Christ has welcomed you, for the glory of God." Romans 15:7 39

"I myself am satisfied about you, my brothers, that you yourselves are full of goodness, filled with all knowledge and able to instruct one another." Romans 15:14

"Greet one another with a holy kiss. All the churches of Christ greet you." Romans 16:15

"For you were called to freedom, brothers. Only do not use your freedom as an opportunity for the flesh, but through love serve one another." Galatians 5:13

"I therefore, a prisoner of the LORD, urge you to walk in a manner worthy of the calling to which you have been called, with all humility and gentleness, with patience, bearing one another in love..." Ephesians 4:1-3

"Be kind to one another, tenderhearted, forgiving one another, as God in Christ forgave you." Ephesians 4:31-32

"...Addressing one another in psalms and hymns and spiritual songs, singing and making melody to the LORD with your heart." Ephesians 5:19

"Submitting to one another out of reverence for Christ." Ephesians 5:21

"Bearing with one another and, if one has a complaint against another, forgiving each other, as the LORD has forgiven you, so you also must forgive." Colossians 3:13

"Let the word of Christ dwell in you richly, teaching and admonishing one another in all wisdom, singing psalms and hymns and spiritual songs, with thankfulness in your hearts to God." Colossians 3:16

"Therefore encourage one another and build one another up, just as you are doing." 1 Thessalonians 5:11

"But exhort one another every day, as long as it is called "today," that none of you may be hardened by the deceitfulness of sin." Hebrews 3:13

"And let us consider how to stir up one another to love and good works, not neglecting to meet together, as is the habit of some, but encouraging one another, and all the more as you see the Day drawing near." Hebrews 10:24-25

"Having purified your souls by your obedience to the truth for a sincere brotherly love, love one another earnestly, from a pure heart." 1 Peter 1:22

"Show hospitality to one another without grumbling." 1 Peter 4:9 41

"Clothe yourselves, all of you, with humility toward one another, for "God opposes the proud but gives grace to the humble." 1 Peter 5:5

"But if we walk in the light, as he is in the light, we have fellowship with one another, and the blood of Jesus His Son cleanses us from all sin." 1 John 1:7

"And this is his commandment, that we believe in the name of his Son Jesus Christ and love one another, just as he has commanded us." 1 John 3:23

"Beloved, if God so loved us, we also ought to love one another. No one has ever seen God; if we love one another, God abides in us and his love is perfected in us." 1 John 4:11-12

"And now I ask you, dear lady—not as though I were writing you a new commandment, but the one we have had from the beginning—that we love one another." 2 John 1:5

VIII
Women Mentoring Women

Women long to experience hospitality and service with their friends and family—within their homes, especially—though often much of that is lost in today's society. Blessing God's Way works as a catalyst to restore these valued virtues to women and families. Each aspect of our ministry gives the opportunity for women to serve other women. Taking the Titus 2 model, women in each "branch", or season of womanhood, can work to help others. BGW would like to facilitate the growth of mentoring relationships between women.

> *"But as for you, teach what accords with sound doctrine. Older men are to be sober-minded, dignified, self-controlled, sound in faith, in love, and in steadfastness. Older women likewise are to be reverent in behavior, not slanderers or slaves to much wine. They are to teach what is good, and so to train the young women to love their husbands and children, to be self-controlled, pure, working at home, kind, and submissive to their own husbands, that the word of God may not be reviled. Likewise, urge the younger men to be self-controlled. Show yourself in all respects to be a model of good works, and in your teaching show integrity, dignity, and sound speech that cannot be condemned, so that an opponent*

may be put to shame, having nothing evil to say about us." Titus 2:1-8

Method to Mentoring

"'Encourage' is the Greek word *sophronizo*. It means 'to recall one to his senses, to admonish (warn), to exhort, to spur on.'"

- Martha Peace, ***Becoming a Titus 2 Woman***

In the Bible, Hebrews speaks about a gathering together to encourage one another: "And let us consider how to stir up one another to love and good works..." Hebrews 10:24 This is one more major area of the Christian church in which we are slacking. It is one more area where we, as Christians, could improve and be set apart unto Him. I will now explain how and by what means this is happening.

The scriptures in Titus 2:1-8 mention that older women should admonish the younger women to do and be many things, all of which are virtuous like self-control, purity, homemakers, kindness, etc. This is a formal "call" to older women to seek and teach and/or disciple the younger generation. This means us—yes, us! We should not say, "I do not know how I am supposed to take on this mentoring role," but rather ask, "Where do I begin and what tools are available to me so that I may start in the process of mentoring women?"

Susan Hunt, from ***Spiritual Mothering***, has said it most beautifully, *"We must not allow the world to set the agenda for this decade, and we must not allow those voices to teach women how to be women."* She also states so eloquently, *"Christian women must speak with boldness and clarity about womanhood and must live distinctly Christian lives."* Oh, this is so true, don't you agree? We have a job to do, in particular, mentoring women through their cycles. We are to:

- Steer women to see God's design for them, particularly as women.
- Encourage women to give thanks and embrace (biblically) their God-given designs as women.
- Give women an outlet or "means" to unveil their gifts for being servers and helpers.
- Offer particular workshops or times to teach about God's design for their cycles (time permitting.)
- Offer hope and encouragement to women of the next generation so they may obtain His understanding of what their cycles were created to be.
- Create awareness that our cycles are not to be feared or dreaded.
- Set an example to the secular world by being Christ-centered, even in our cycles.
- Pray for one another and serve one another.

The absolute awesome and beautiful thing about this whole concept and implementation of the Mentoring Program in your community is that it does not necessarily have to be a "church" function or through a church entity. I believe it will have to come from passionate mothers who see the need for this type of mentoring relationship to happen. If your church supports the Blessing God's Way mission, we can equip you with the tools you will need to begin a church ministry in the way of mentoring, though it doesn't have to be through a church, per se.

Begin mentoring in your neck of the woods. Stop dreaming about it. Stop complaining that there aren't enough women to do it, but instead pray about how you can take advantage of the tools available to you. It is all about faith. Pick up your foot, while not knowing where it will be set down, and trust it will be set down ever so gently by our loving Father and that He may bless the fruit of your labor in doing so.

Do's and Don'ts of Mentoring

Mentor Do's	Mentor Don'ts
Praise the mentee when deserved	Don't judge the mentee
Appreciate any growth	Don't think you can change the world overnight
Ask questions and gather information	Don't forget that confidence is built on trust
Be punctual	Dont' disappoint a mentee that's counting on you by being late in correspondence
Be a good role model	Don't use inappropriate language (oral or written)
Follow the scriptures at all times	Don't allow mentees to talk you into things that are against scripture
Show attention and concern by being a freind	Don't try to be an authority in a high position

Do's and Don'ts of Mentoring

Mentor Do's	Mentor Don'ts
Recognize the mentees values and lifestyles	Don't impose your beliefs or values on the mentee, but demonstrate your Christ-likeness
Share with the mentee and communicate	Don't forget that communication means listening
Strive for mutual respect	Don't tolerate rudeness or disrespect
Be prepared	Don't mentor without a plan
Be honest	Don't think a mentee can't spot insincerity
Assist the mentee	Don't do the work of change for the mentee
Encourage and uplift	Don't berate or belittle
Be a coach and motivator	Don't serve as a social worker or professional counselor

IX

Resting in the Lord

When you are experiencing your first cycle in maidenhood, you are embarking on a new phase in your life as a woman. God has called you to have this cycle for about 40 years and to use it as a cleansing time for you while your body is not carrying a child. Your time of the month has come, and your body is feeling the aches and pains of the weeks previous. Your mind, body, and spirit are working overtime to keep a loving attitude for those around you. You long to have a moment to yourself for thoughts and prayers.

Perhaps, in maternity, you are overwhelmed with all the new sensations your body is experiencing with growth and hormonal activity. You have rejoiced with the LORD at the wonder of first hearing your baby's heartbeat, seeing him/her for the first time during a sonogram, and feeling the first kick. His grace was sufficient through the trials of morning sickness, your belly stretching beyond what you could have imagined, never-ending heartburn, and those baby aerobics in the wee hours of the morning. Maybe you have lost so much sleep during the transition of your hormones playing all night that your spirit is tired and not sure how it will continue.

In menopause, the time has come for you to look at life without the regular cycle that you have known. You are knee-deep in new sensations and activity happening in your life, not only when you least expect it, but also when it is most likely unwelcome. You are dealing with the realization that you cannot bear children anymore, and your life is changing. Enduring the changes is stressful and complicated, but you want to endure and conqueror this phase with a positive outlook and by being an example to those around you.

The good news is that God's grace continues. Although we acknowledge all things happen in His time, we often find ourselves asking for His time to move faster. Now are the seasons when God wants us to lean more steadfastly on Him. Through our cycles, we are to rest in Him. Lay it all at the foot of the cross and feel His arms place our faces heavenward, from whence comes our help.

> *"Come to me, all who labor and are heavy laden, and I will give you rest. Take my yoke upon you, and learn from me, for I am gentle and lowly in heart, and you will find rest for your souls. For my yoke is easy, and my burden is light."* Matthew 11:28-30

Savor a Moment of Rest:

- Keep a Bible next to your bed and when you wake in the morning, vow to read a Psalm to start your day.

- Start a practice of gentle yoga stretches and breath with movement.

- Gather a candle and praise and worship music, then close the door to your bathroom to take a warm bath for at least 10 minutes.

- Start a journal, writing your prayers and supplications with thanksgiving to the LORD our

God, for the upcoming transition in your household. Take time each day to add to this journal.

- Seek out encouragement from women who are experienced with the cycle you are in, or for motherhood and childbirth, which will give you emotional support.

- Share with your mother, trusted friend, and/or husband the beautiful aspects of Christ and His blessings and how you can both rejoice in this phase.

- Seek out other Godly people who have experienced what you are experiencing, get the benefit of their knowledge.

- Exercise well and maintain a great diet. This alone will lift your spirits and give you a feeling of refreshment and rest.

- Go take a walk in the sun. Sunlight is great medicine and a motivator to be rejuvenated.

X

Celebration Gatherings

As you read in the introduction to this book, I created a gathering that celebrates pregnancy and childbirth. We have called it a *Blessing God's Way* gathering or a *Celebration of Pregnancy* gathering. Maidenhood and menopause can be celebrated as well, with a lot of the same elements as the pregnancy gathering. The point of these is to help steer women to God, to His goodness, mercy, and design. The celebrations (formally known as Blessingways) can simply be called Celebration Gatherings. They are used as an opportunity to gather, so that we can give thanks, praise God, and uplift and encourage our fellow women in all phases of womanhood.

I am placing here a step-by-step section for you to use next time you have an opportunity to serve a friend or family member by celebrating the onset of their first cycle beginning, the gift of their child, or the waning of their cycle. When a young woman begins her cycle, consider having a few very close friends over with their mothers and have a special gathering to teach them to see God in their lives for this season. For maternity, you can celebrate the new life for this family and give her encouragement and inspiration to see God's honor bestowed upon her in the gift of their child. When a woman reaches menopause, life has shifted and moved in a different direction. That change can be acknowledged and honored for her. A Celebration Gathering is a great opportunity to recognize the changes, supporting her through the transition that sometimes can be very drastic or span over a few years.

Our culture has misguided pictures of what these seasons are supposed to be in our lives, but celebrating with a Celebration Gathering provides us with a way to be a good example, shining light into the darkness that is often so prevalent. Having a Celebration Gathering allows the hostess to exercise her gifts of hospitality and service towards others. It allows the guest of honor to take time out of her busy life, as well as to provide a time of joy and fellowship to the guests and the one who is hosting.

Why celebrate? First and foremost, we want to give honor, glory, and praise to our God for His gift, no matter which cycle or phase we are in. Secondly, we want to bring women and families together to celebrate and give support to the honored guest in their new season of life.

The word blessing means "a short prayer for divine approval." To bless a mother, we are invoking God's favor upon her for her "way," the journey, and through her transition ahead. Women need support and encouragement throughout their seasons, and having a Celebration Gathering provides this through scripture reading, praise to our LORD, singing of songs, and partaking in a meal together.

Before continuing on, please remember that a Celebration Gathering is an avenue for women and families to come together to give honor to God for either the onset of menstruation for their daughter or loved one, for the gift of a child, or for the blessing of menopause when our cycle ceases to exist, and we begin a new phase in life. By encouraging celebrations for pregnancy, we are not advocating any particular point of view in the area of family planning. Each of us has our own relationship with the LORD, and we walk out our paths differently. The Blessing God's Way ministry teaches a simpler message, that God is the Giver and Creator of menstruation, children, and our cycles ending, and that they all are a blessing.

Material List

Below you will find a list of materials that we hope will be helpful in planning a Celebration Gathering. Feel free to gather the materials yourself.

- Hairbrush
- Hair ties, pins
- Dried or real flowers
- Very warm water
- Basin for a foot bath
- Lighter or matches
- Box of tissues
- Pillows
- Towel
- Soothing music
- Invitations
- Games
- Sand for a tray of candles
- Candles for the tray of sand
- Herbs for foot wash
- Massage oil for massage
- Tea light candles or ask guests to bring them
- This book for reproducible materials and resources to share
- Beads to create necklaces or bracelets
- Henna powder (organic and from a reputable source) for temporary tattoos
- Scripture cards (made or purchased)

Special Surroundings

We all have those favorite areas in our home where we can unwind and feel relaxed. For the Celebration Gathering, we want to create that area for her, as well as add an extra amount of comfort to the surroundings, if possible. The honored guest needs a place where she can see all the "pretties" around her, where she can feel joy and happiness by simply looking around the room. A suggestion would be to touch the five senses in some manner:

- Get out special cloths or spreads to stretch out on the ground where you will gather;

- Fill the room with fresh flowers from the outdoors;

- Have candles burning to create a light that is pleasing and welcoming;

- Depending on the weather, use the outdoors to have fresh air blowing and crisp air to breathe;

- Make sure all the chairs, spreads, and pillows are soft and smooth to the touch;

- Have spiritual and encouraging music playing softly in the background.

Sample Songs for *Blessingways*

We have included songs, in the Resource section in Chapter 11, that we feel will allow you to give praise and honor to God for His blessing to the honored guest. The songs also offer encouragement, inspiration, and exhortation during this time in her life. Please feel free to copy them (they may need to be enlarged) and distribute them to your guests.

> *"I will sing of steadfast love and justice; to You, O LORD, I will make music."* Psalm 101:1

> *"Is anyone among you suffering? Let him pray. Is anyone cheerful? Let him sing praise."* James 5:13

"Let the word of Christ dwell in you richly, teaching and admonishing one another in all wisdom, singing psalms and hymns and spiritual songs, with thankfulness in your hearts to God." Colossians 3:16

Fellowship Meal

At the closing of a Celebration Gathering, the guests are asked to gather and partake in a meal together. Sharing fellowship with one another is part of this celebration. Always remember our food is from Him and of Him. We are being filled with the bread of life! One of the benefits of Jesus dying on the cross is that we can entertain and share a fellowship meal with our loved ones. Food is a blessing. It is also nourishing, sustaining, and life-giving.

"Bread is made for laughter..." Ecclesiastes 10:19

"...But the cheerful of heart has a continual feast." Proverbs 15:15

For women having a baby or who are going through menopause, you can use this food train sign up list to encourage meal trains for their time of transition. There are plenty of online resources to do this electronically, as well.

Additional Tips & Suggestions

Over the years, I have received so many suggestions and tips for celebrating. I hope these are helpful as you put together your Celebration Gathering.

Breaking bread with one another in a fellowship meal is an intimate gesture. It should be sweet and lasting (not in a hurry to get everyone out and home when the clock strikes 2:00). We don't mean to say that you should keep everyone in your home all day, either, of course! Have a schedule for the Celebration Gathering, but don't be too harsh in sticking to the minute of it. Remember, we want to make a statement of "relax" to our honored guest and friends.

A Celebration Gathering is an intimate gathering for close friends and loved ones. When you make your invitation list, make sure you include people who are comfortable around one another. Of course, everyone present does not have to be a Christian. We pray that by hearing the word of God at this gathering, their hearts will be turned to Him. We know that scripture does not come back void.

When inviting women and young ladies to a Celebration Gathering, consider inviting husbands and other children to take part in this celebration. In some instances, this would be appropriate, but in other instances, it wouldn't. Remember, this is a time for the honored guest to relax, and sometimes having little children around would defeat that purpose. The focus should be first on the LORD, then on the honored guest, and then on the rest of the family/friends present. If this is for a celebration of pregnancy, you can also invite their midwives or physicians, giving them an opportunity to get to know their clients better.

When scheduling a pregnancy Celebration Gathering, remember to do it close to the due date, but not too close. We want to give her this relaxation toward the end, but remember she may go two weeks early or two weeks late. This is when it is most appreciated by the mother-to-be. For a menses or menopause Celebration Gathering, you have more leeway and can schedule it when the time is appropriate to really minister to her soul. We have had women host a Celebration Gathering after a baby is born, or for a stillbirth, or a miscarriage, to honor the fact that the mother had been pregnant, and God bestowed a child to them for a time. This takes delicate discernment, so please pray over this type of celebration.

The host or another guest could start a scrapbook with all the poems, blessings, and thoughts that were presented at the gathering. The honored guest would then have the scrapbook, which she may like to look at while she is in her time of month, in labor, or going through menopause. This can be very encouraging to her. A Celebration Gathering scrapbook paper album is available for this occasion. This can be purchased from Blessing God's Way online, or you can purchase a plain one from your favorite store.

Taking and printing photos from the Celebration Gathering will be an awesome addition to the scrapbook when completed. Having the photos to view will be a treat and joy for the honored guest and her family for years to come. This book can be given to the honored guest after the gathering. It includes prayers and scriptures that can be referenced easily by her for the rest of her cycles and beyond.

Some women enjoy making a prayer bracelet or necklace for the honored guest. You can do this by asking everyone to bring a bead, and with it, they can give their "gift from the heart." The young lady, mother, or menopausal woman could wear this in remembrance of the women or ladies who stand behind her and who have gone before her.

Henna has become a popular way of expressing love and community, especially as a reassurance that you have a "tribe" who supports you in the season of life you are in. You can look into having henna designs done either on the guest of honor only (hand, belly, feet), or everyone can have a small design created. Be aware not to use cheap, black henna ink, which can cause side effects from the chemicals used. Instead, purchase organic henna powder from a reputable resource.

If you are hosting this Celebration Gathering for adopting parents or parents who have experienced loss, consider being more mindful and sensitive to the family you serve. Families who adopt have gone through a vigorous process to finally obtain official papers and custody, so we want to honor them for enduring that process and give God glory for it. For those who have had a loss, a Celebration Gathering can be used to recognize that this mom was pregnant, and there still is a baby to be celebrated. It is a tool to help a mom process the grief and share her story as she continues to heal.

You can have quoted scripture on big paper hung on the walls in the room where the women will be meeting and celebrating, as a reminder to hide His word in our hearts. The honored guest can then take the scriptures home as a keepsake and re-tape them on her walls for extra help focusing on God's goodness to her. Affirmation Cards are also wonderful encouragement and reminders.

Basic Instructional Outline for a Celebration Gathering

Choose either an indoor or outdoor special place to host the Celebration Gathering. You will need the materials from the kit. Go out of your way to make the surroundings as inviting and pretty as you can (see Special Surroundings in Part One).

Gather the group in a circle. At this time, you can introduce yourself and explain why you have chosen to do a Celebration Gathering (refer to the Blessing God's Way vision and introduction at the beginning of this book).

Offer up a prayer to begin. You could offer thanks to our LORD for the person you are honoring and the transition she is about to go through, for God's goodness in His blessing to her in this phase of life, as well as ask for guidance and strength for her upcoming cycle/s. You could pray over the time spent during the gathering, that it will bring glory to Him who makes all things. (See the sample prayer below or make up your own.)

Sample prayer for opening a Celebration Gathering:

We thank you LORD, for this day, for this time to gather and give you glory for such a great gift as being a woman made by your perfect design. You have made us fearfully and wonderfully, and we know that full well. We are grateful you have called us to come together to support, encourage and uplift this young lady/woman. Give us a humble and serving spirit toward this honored guest. Please bless our time and the people gathered here today. We pray this in Jesus Christ's name, Amen.

Now would be a good time to sing the Doxology, which is a wonderful opening song to give praise and thanks to the LORD. Again, you want to help all the participants to focus on the true reason for such a joyous occasion.

Praise God from Whom all blessings flow,

Praise Him all creatures here below,

Praise Him above ye heavenly host,

Praise Father, Son, and Holy Ghost.

Have all participants introduce themselves and share how they know the honored guest. You could also implement another icebreaker to get everyone relaxed and comfortable.

Let's sing! Singing songs, praise and giving glory to our LORD, is an important part of this gathering. Use the enclosed song sheets to copy (you may have to enlarge) and hand out so that the participants may join their voices together. You could sing a few in the beginning and then another one later, depending on when it would be appropriate, and spread several songs throughout the gathering. If you have favorite songs, please use them in place of the ones we have included in this book. A playlist specifically created for the gathering can be listened to, if you do not feel comfortable in leading the singing. Another idea is to have one of the guests who is gifted in piano or another instrument share their talent, which would be an extra touch of blessing on the Celebration Gathering.

Next, you can share how this gathering is meant to give glory to God for the particular cycle being celebrated. Encourage the honored guest by giving blessings from the heart and words of encouragement and support. You can speak of how God has designed our bodies for our cycles and that His grace is sufficient.

Point out how 40 weeks (the time of gestation for pregnancy and the time a woman menstruates on average) is a number God uses over and over for transitions that bring about great change and blessing. The number 40 is often understood as the "number of probation or trial." For example, the Israelites wandered for 40 years (Deuteronomy 8:2-5); Moses was on the mount for 40 days (Exodus 24:18); 40 days were involved in the story of Jonah and Nineveh (Jonah 3:4); Jesus was tempted for 40 days (Matthew 4:2); there were 40 days between Jesus' resurrection and ascension (Acts 1:3). He describes to us that these times are for testing our hearts and minds, but that, in the end, the "Promised Land" is oh, so sweet to behold, making it all worthwhile!

> *"The whole commandment that I command you today you shall be careful to do, that you may live and multiply, and go in and possess the land that the LORD swore to give your fathers. And you shall remember the whole way that the LORD your God has led you these forty years in the wilderness, that He might humble you, testing you to know what was in your heart, whether you would keep His commandments or not. For the LORD your God is bringing you into a good land, a land of brooks of water, of fountains and springs, flowing out in the valleys and hills; .and you shall bless the LORD your God for the good land which He has given you."* Deuteronomy 8:1-10

Decorate the honored guest's hair with flowers (fresh, dried, fabric, fake). Having the younger girls braid and brush her hair is very touching, and they really enjoy this part. You could also make a crown of flowers, putting that on her when her hair is finished being brushed or braided. Don't forget to take pictures!

Next, you can get a bowl filled with warm/hot water and pour in the herbs with a few drops of massage oil (almond, coconut or olive oil is preferred). Make sure you have plenty of towels nearby. Let the honored guest soak her feet for a few minutes (a good time to sing or play a song). Have her mother wash her feet (if present), then the mother-in-law, sisters, or best friends. Open it up to whoever would like to participate. Singing another song here would be nice. Talk about how this is an ultimate gesture of humility and service toward one another as it may be uncomfortable for both. Nonetheless, it is a spiritual experience you will not forget easily. Most women who are unsure about this portion usually exclaim how wonderful it was to do or to have it done to them. It brings a feeling of vulnerability, but one of complete servanthood as well.

> *"If I then, your Lord and Teacher, have washed your feet,*
> *you also ought to wash one another's feet."* John 13:14

Massage the feet with the foot massage oil. Ask for others to come and help. You might also want to massage her hands, just to give the honored guest a little extra pampering. Massage is medicinal, promoting circulation in the body and reducing swelling and aches.

> *"Oil and perfume make the heart glad."* Proverbs 27:9

Now is the time to light candles. Share any special handmade gifts, poems, blessings, or thoughts for encouragement. The lighting of candles is simply used to remind us that the LORD is our Light and gives us light. One person lights her candle and gives her a gift from the heart, then the next person in the circle does the same. A gift from the heart can be a drawing, scripture, or anything that comes from the heart with meaning and love.

> *"The LORD is my light and my salvation; whom shall I*
> *fear? The LORD is the stronghold of my life; of whom*
> *shall I be afraid?"* Psalm 27:1

Explain to the honored guest that she can re-light these candles when she starts her period that month, goes into labor, or when she is having a very bad menopause day. She then can be reminded of all those gathered at the Celebration Gathering and how they are supporting her in spirit.

Have the first person light a candle, place it in the tray, then present their words and/or blessing, advice, or drawing (gift from the heart). The next person lights a candle and does the same. Continue all the way around the circle.

Once all the prayers, blessings, and poems are gathered, give them to the honored guest with a scrapbook for her to make a keepsake. Or, as suggested previously, give a scrapbook and contents to the guest who volunteered to compile it.

> *"In all things I have shown that by working hard in this way we must help the weak and remember the words of the LORD Jesus, how he himself said, "It is more blessed to give than to receive." Acts 20:35*

> *"For you were called to freedom, brothers. Only do not use your freedom as an opportunity for the flesh, but through love serve one another. For the whole law is fulfilled in one word: `You shall love your neighbor as yourself.'" Galatians 5:13-14*

Now would be a good time to present the gift certificate if you have compiled contributions for this. A gift card or certificate would be useful as a treat or to save for a rainy day. For an expecting mother, it can be used to get exactly what she needs for that particular pregnancy. (See section on Gift Certificates & Gift Cards)

Finally, pray again, laying hands on the honored woman, asking a blessing on the food you are about to partake, and for a blessing upon the honored guest. Invite everyone to stay and eat and be merry!

"And I commend joy, for man has nothing better under the sun but to eat and drink and be joyful, for this will go with him in his toil through the days of his life that God has given him under the sun." Ecclesiastes 8:15

Introduce the concept of a Food Train Sign Up. This can be for bringing meals to a woman after having her baby, for a woman dealing with difficult menopause symptoms, or even for a young lady to spark some light in her life and uplift her with food that she enjoys! Only the pregnancy sign up would require a week's worth of meals, while the other cycles and phases of womanhood could use maybe once a month or when appropriate.

Gift Certificate Options

Having guests contribute to a gift certificate is an option for a gift-giving idea instead of having the traditional "opening of gifts." Gift certificates or cards are especially nice to show you have taken an extra amount of care in blessing the honored guest. Be sure to include this idea on the invitation sent out to the invited guests.

XI

Resources

In this next section, you will find poems, Scriptures, prayers, and songs that you can use during a Celebration Gathering.

The copyrighted songs and poems in this section may only be used for a Celebration Gathering. Using the songs and poems for any other purpose requires permission from the copyright owner(s). We appreciate your honesty in this matter.

The following names are the authors of the copyrighted songs and poems we have gathered for this guide: Shelly Stockton, *Lead Me & May the Words*; Melissa Taylor, *The Voice of the Lord*; Doran Richards, *Gift from God*; Rachel Himelright, *Blessing;* Janet Miller, *Motherhood 101*

Any of the resources on the following pages can be gifts from the heart that you can use during your *Celebration Gathering*. Please feel free to copy and give this to the guest of honor for her scrapbook or for remembrance of this special time in her life.

Maidenhood Resources

POEMS & QUOTES

I'd Rather See a Sermon
by Edgar A. Guest

I'd rather see a sermon than hear one any day,
I'd rather one should walk with me than merely tell the way.
The eye's a better pupil and more willing than the ear,
Fine counsel is confusing, but example's always clear;
And the best of all the preachers are the men who live their creeds,
For to see good put in action is what everybody needs.
I soon can learn to do it if you'll let me see it done;
I can watch your hands in action, but your tongue too fast may run.
And the lecture you deliver may be very wise and true,
But I'd rather get my lessons by observing what you do;
For I might misunderstand you and the high advice you give,
But there's no misunderstanding how you act and how you live.

"Every day, our girl will meet with circumstances in which she has her choice between frowning and sending back a stinging retort, or smiling and passing them by with a kind word. If she can pass these little bumps and keep sweet, then she has mastered the art of being sunny."

- Mabel Hale , **Beautiful Girlhood**

"Live in the sunshine. Look on the bright side, for there is always a bright side."

- Mabel Hale , **Beautiful Girlhood**

"All women are born with the need to communicate at a deeper level with their mothers, grandmothers, sisters, daughters, aunts, cousins, and other significant females in their lives. Wholesome friendships among women promote sound mental and emotional health. Friends remind us we are part of something greater than our selves, a larger world, and the right friends keep us on track. Now is the time to reclaim and re-establish ourselves as friends."

- Barbara Jenkins, **Wit and Wisdom for Women**

SCRIPTURE ENCOURAGEMENT

"And my God will supply every need of yours according to His riches in glory in Christ Jesus." Philippians 4:19

"But He said to me, "My grace is sufficient for you, for my power is made perfect in weakness." Therefore I will boast all the more gladly of my weakness, so that the power of Christ may rest upon me. For the sake of Christ, then, I am content with weakness, insults, hardships,

persecutions, and calamities. For when I am weak, then I am strong." 2 Corinthians 12:9-10

"But they who wait for the LORD shall renew their strength; they shall mount up with wings like eagles; they shall run and not be weary; they shall walk and not faint." Isaiah 40:31

"And let us not grow weary of doing good, for in due season we will reap, if we do not give up." Galatians 6:9

"If any of you lacks wisdom, let him ask God, who gives generously to all without reproach, and it will be given to him." James 1:5

"He who calls you is faithful; he will surely do it." 1 Thessalonians 5:24

"If we confess our sins, He is faithful and just to forgive us our sins and to cleanse us from all unrighteousness." 1 John 1:9

"Oh give thanks to the LORD, for He is good, for His steadfast love endures forever!" Psalm 107:1

"Give thanks in all circumstances; for this is the will of God in Christ Jesus for you." 1 Thessalonians 5:18

"I will sing to the LORD, because He has dealt bountifully with me." Psalm 13:6

"...Great is your faithfulness." Lamentations 3:23

INSPIRATIONAL ARTICLE

10 Steps to Mastering Your Thoughts and Moods
by Rebecca Chamaa

Like the old saying goes, "Which came first, the chicken or the egg?" which came first for us, the negative thought or the foul mood? No matter which did, the two go hand in hand. You can become a master at controlling your thoughts and moods by practicing these ten exercises. You can also fulfill this passage from scripture at the same time:

"We destroy arguments and every lofty opinion raised against the knowledge of God, and take every thought captive to obey Christ..." 2 Corinthians 10:5

1. Memorize this passage of Scripture and put it into practice:

   "Finally, brothers, whatever is true, whatever is honorable, whatever is just, whatever is pure, whatever is lovely, whatever is commendable, if there is any excellence, if there is anything worthy of praise, think about these things." Philippians 4:8

2. Another good way to halt and change the direction of negative thoughts and bad moods is to stop and begin to thank God for all that is good or right in your life. It is hard to be in a bad mood or have negative thoughts when you start to list your blessings. Depending upon the severity of the mood, a short list will probably start to lift your spirits, but if it doesn't, try listing the things we often overlook. Dig deep in your heart for what you might have that others long to have (eyesight, hearing, food, clothes, shelter, the ability to walk or bend over, joints that don't ache, etc.).

3. Start a hope list. Think about all that you would like to have happen over the coming year and write it down. Next, think about all the things you would like to have happened over

the next six months and write them down. Make a list of the things you would like to have happen in the next month and write them down. Pick one item from each list and write steps that you can take to make these things a reality. Pray about your hope list and visit it often to make changes, mark progress, and add steps to help you accomplish these things.

4. Another way to change the course of your thoughts is to stop and ask God to take control of your day. Just give the day over to God and let Him know you need His help. This usually provides some much-needed comfort and the hope that things will begin to change.

5. Taking action is an effective way to lift your spirits. It could be as simple as taking action against a dirty house (if you do this one, start with one room, and start with a small chore first so you can see your progress), or it could be starting to work on a project that has been sitting for a long time, or it could be writing a letter. The possibilities for this exercise are endless.

6. Take a walk and use the time to either talk to God, or listen to an audio sermon, the Bible on tape, or Christian music. The walk alone should help give your mood a boost, and the time spent worshiping will be an added lift.

7. Write down all the negative thoughts you are having and then spend some time looking through the Bible for verses that oppose your thoughts. A quick and easy way to do this is by buying a book that addresses everyday problems with Scriptures. I recommend *God's Promises for Every Day*, by A.L. Gill, the New Century Version.

8. Say the Lord's Prayer over and over again until you can get through it without having any other thoughts intrude (you might find that you have to say it up to ten times). Start over every time you catch your mind wandering.

9. Think about the people you know and the struggles they are having, or think about people in parts of the world and their struggles. Stop and say a prayer for all those you thought about.

10. Sing your favorite Christian song from beginning to end. Keep singing it until you start to feel better.

If you try all ten exercises, and you find that you still can't shake those negative thoughts or a bad mood, then keep in mind that the real Master is always there to assist you and with His help and guidance you will be tapped into the ultimate source of joy and strength.

You can also call everyone you know and let them know that God created both the chicken and the egg, and the mystery is just His way of "fowling" around!

© *by Rebecca Chamaa. Used with permission.*

About the Author: Rebecca was a social worker in Washington State for over seven years. Five of those years were spent working with Children and Family Services. She currently lives in Southern California with her husband.

RECOMMENDED BOOKS

Maidens by His Design Teacher's Guide by Doran Richards
Maidens by His Design Student Workbook by Doran Richards
(available on Amazon)

Lady Day: Letters to a Daughter About Becoming a Woman by Joy Moore

Beautifully Made by Generations of Virtue

God's Plan for Growing Up, From Girl...To Woman! by Sandi Queen

RECOMMENDED WEBSITES

Aviva Romm, MD
www.avivaromm.com

Blessing God's Way - Doran Richards
www.blessinggodsway.com

The Period Revolution - Laura Briden
www.laurabriden.com

Maternity Resources

POEMS

Gift from God
by Doran Richards © 2001

I give thanks to You alone
Who sits on the throne.
To loan me this precious gift
And to call it my own.

May I always see, Lord
In every waking hour,
Your majesty and grace
In this delicate flower.

Help me, O God,
To guide and preserve,
This wonderful blessing
To love and to serve.

Blessing
by Rachel Himelright © 2004

The blessing of a child is the biggest jewel.
How indescribable is it to look into the face of your
newborn baby?
How can words speak the joy and pain and beauty
of seeing your child grow?
How can the finite be used to describe the feelings
that run the gamut of the infinite?
God blesses this way, and the world scorns it.

The devil hates the gift of a child.

The devil seeks to destroy as many as he can, and corrupt the ones that live.

The devil seeks to lie and cheat so many of the joy of this gift.

So many buy into his agenda, going to great lengths to avoid God's greatest gift

Not so, you.

You have sought His face, and time and again he has blessed you.

You have seen the heartache of pain and have felt those emotions that words can not describe.

You have touched the face of your children and perhaps seen there the closest thing to heaven on this earth.

You have seen something so shrouded in mystery that even having seen it, you cannot describe its beauty, God's blessing.

God's blessing and you are the instrument of its arrival.

Through this child, God provides an opportunity for us to see a picture of His relationship with us.

Through this child, God provides your family with a lifetime of a deep and meaningful relationship.

Through this child, God forever alters the landscape of your life, and adds to it, creating a fullness never found in the empty philosophies of this world.

A touch of heaven in your hands.

A touch of the Father in your keeping.

A touch of the greatest mystery for you to kiss.

No matter how the world tries to explain it away and demonize it, God has ordained the gift of life as His

blessing, His heritage, His beautiful picture
I ache for those who have missed it.
Some even in our family disdain the beauty and
wonder of the child and what it means.

Only God can spark the life that is our soul.
Only a conception He ordained can bring everything
together just so.
Only we were created using His breath and hands.

The rest He spoke, but for us He crafted,
His modeling in His image, Body, Soul, and Spirit.
And still this day He knits, forming us in the womb
because He loves us.

Longing for our hearts, He chases us, and brings us
full circle, letting us witness the mystery that is a
baby, so we can glimpse His love for us at creation
and still.

Little People
by John Greenleaf Whittier

A dreary place would be this earth
Were there no little people in it;
The Song of life would lose its mirth,
Were there no children to begin it.

No little forms, like buds to grow,
And make the admiring heart surrender
No little hands on breast and brow,
To Keep the thrilling love-chords tender.

The sterner souls would grow more stern,
Unfeeling nature more inhuman,
And man to stoic coldness turn,
And Woman would be less than woman.

Life's song, indeed, would lose its charm,
Were there no babies to begin it;
A doleful place this world would be,
Were there no little people in it.

Be Thou My Vision
Irish poem translated by Elizabeth Byrne -1905

Be Thou my Vision, O Lord of my heart;
Naught be all else to me, save that Thou art

Thou my best Thought, by day or by night,
Waking or sleeping, Thy presence my light.

Be Thou my Wisdom, and Thou my true Word;
I ever with Thee and Thou with me, Lord;

Thou my great Father, I Thy true son;
Thou in me dwelling, and I with Thee one.

Be Thou my battle Shield, Sword for the fight;

Be Thou my Dignity, Thou my Delight;

Thou my soul's Shelter, Thou my high Tower:
Raise Thou me heavenward, O Power of my power.

Riches I heed not, nor man's empty praise,
Thou mine Inheritance, now and always:

Thou and Thou only, first in my heart,
High King of heaven, my Treasure Thou art.

High King of heaven, my victory won,
May I reach heaven's joys, O bright heaven's Sun!

Heart of my own heart, whatever befall,
Still be my Vision, O Ruler of all.

SCRIPTURES & PRAYERS

"Be anxious for nothing, but in everything by prayer and supplication, with thanksgiving, let your requests be made known to God; and the peace of God, which surpasses all understanding, will guard your hearts and minds through Christ Jesus." Philippians 4:6-7

On the Coming of a New Baby
from the Book of Prayer (Mother's Prayer)

Lord Jesus Christ, Thou Good Shepherd who dost delight in the little babes and dost gently lead those that are with young, I thank Thee for Thy marvelous mercy. Thou hast granted my husband and me the gift of a healthy child, and I cannot praise Thee enough for Thy loving-kindness. Thou hast guided the physician, given me strength during my pregnancy and delivery, and sustained me to this moment.

Give me a grateful heart all the days of my life, and enable me to be the kind of mother who will please Thee. Keep me conscious at all times of the holy trust placed in me by the gift of this child, and help me to bring my child up in Thy fear and favor.

Send Thy guardian angels to watch over my little one, and shield him/her from all danger of body or soul. Take my child into Thy kingdom, and give him/her an inheritance with all Thy saints.

Oh, Thou who hast given life to my child, be Thou our Good Shepherd, and lead us in paths pleasing to Thee. Amen.

Need of Jesus
by Puritan Prayers & Devotions,
The Valley of Vision

Lord Jesus,

I am blind, be thou my light,
    ignorant, be thou my wisdom,
    self-willed, be thou my mind.

Open my ear to grasp quickly thy Spirit's voice,
    and delightfully run after his beckoning hand;

Melt my conscience that no hardness remain,
    make it alive to evil's slightest touch;

When Satan approaches may I flee to thy wounds,
    and there cease to tremble at all alarms.

Be my good shepherd to lead me into
    the green pastures of thy Word,
    and cause me to lie down beside the rivers
    of its comforts.

Fill me with peace, that no disquieting worldly gales
    may ruffle the calm surface of my soul.

Thy cross was upraised to be my refuge,

Thy blood streamed forth to wash me clean,

Thy death occurred to give me a surety,

Thy name is my property to save me,

By thee, all heaven is poured into my heart,
    but it is too narrow to comprehend thy love.

I was a stranger, an outcast, a slave, a rebel,
    but thy cross has brought me near,
    has softened my heart
    has made me thy Father's child,
    has admitted me to thy family,
    has made me joint-heir with thyself.

O that I may love thee as thou lovest me,
    that I may walk worthy of thee, my LORD,
    that I may reflect the image of heaven's first-born.

May I always see thy beauty with the clear eye of faith,
    and feel the power of thy Spirit in my heart,
    for unless He moves mightily in me,
    no inward fire will be kindled.

RECOMMENDED BOOKS

Angel in the Water by Regina Doman

Be Fruitful and Multiply by Nancy Campbell

Christ Centered Childbirth by Kelly J. Townsend

Culpeper's Book of Birth Edited and Intro by Ian Thomas

LORD of Birth by Jennifer VanderLaan

40 Weeks Devotional Guide to Pregnancy by Jennifer Vanderlaan

Meditations for the New Mother by Helen Good Brenneman

Mommy Diagnostics by Shonda Parker

Naturally Healthy Pregnancy by Shonda Parker

Prayers for Expectant Mothers by Angela Thomas Guffey

The Christian Childbirth Handbook by Jennifer Vanderlaan

The Ministry of Midwifery by Patti Barnes

RECOMMENDED WEBSITES

Charis Childbirth Services
www.charischildbirth.org

In His Hands Birth Supplies
www.inhishands.com

Childbirth Education
www.childbirtheducation.org

Childbirth Connection
www.childbirthconnection.org

VBAC Facts - Jen Kamel
www.vbacfacts.com

Evidence Based Birth - Rebecca Dekker
www.evidencebasedbirth.com

Ministry of Midwifery - Patti Barnes
www.ministryofmidwifery.com

Grace Midwifery - Doran Richards
www.gracemidwifery.com

Menopause Resources

QUOTES & EXCERPTS

"After the glorious years of childbearing, a wonderful season of life, called menopause occurs. It is a marking of the passing of fertility into feminine maturity. The cycle begins to depart, and a new myriad of hormones will fluctuate wildly until settling down for the remaining years of your life. This is not a time of dread or unhappiness, but one of rejoicing over the years full of bringing life into the world and now perhaps on becoming a grandmother to the greatest joys you will most likely ever experience."
- ***Marvelous Menopause*** by Kristi Zittle of His Grace Herbals (www.hisgraceherbals.com)

"Laughter brings us closer to people, moves us into more positive mind-sets, can stimulate our immune system, enhance our learning and memory, and help us cope better with the stressors in our lives."
- ***Laugh*** by Leslee Kagan, MS, FNP

"Even if the whole earth worships at the temple of youth, do we—and millions of other smart, seasoned, spiritual women like us—really have to be age-a-phobic?"

"If such great care was taken in Old Testament times to build and maintain God's tabernacle, how much more should we care for our bodies, which are God's living, holy temples?"

"It's easy to look in the mirror and obsess about the changing face of our lives. It's more challenging to get still enough to listen and understand what the God Who Never Changes is trying to say to us through it."
- ***Honey, They Shrunk My Hormones*** by Caron Chandler Loveless

Time to Lighten Up

10 Ways to Know if you have Estrogen Issues

1. Everyone around you has an attitude problem.

2. You're adding chocolate chips to your cheese omelet.

3. The dryer has shrunk every last pair of your jeans.

4. Your husband is suddenly agreeing to everything you say.

5. You're using your cellular phone to dial up every bumper sticker that says: "How's my driving-- call 1-800-***."

6. Everyone's head looks like an invitation to batting practice.

7. You're convinced there's a God and he's male.

8. You can't believe they don't make a tampon bigger than Super Plus.

9. You're sure that everyone is scheming to drive you crazy.

10. The ibuprofen bottle is empty and you bought it yesterday.

PRAYERS

A Prayer for Women

Dear Lord,

So far today, I am doing all right. I have not gossiped, lost my temper, been greedy, grumpy, nasty, selfish, or self-

indulgent. *I have not whined, complained, cursed, or eaten any chocolate. I have not charged anything on my credit card. However, I am going to get out of bed in a few minutes, and I will need a lot more help after that. Thanks. Amen.*

New Life
by Pamela M. Smith, R.D. (**When Your Hormones Go Haywire**)

"In any change, there is a golden opportunity to create new life. In this time of "the" change, we can see new life being created in ourselves. We become freer to choose where to direct our efforts and energies. Personal passions and interests burst forth, which many women funnel into new businesses, ministries, careers, volunteerism, or hobbies."

RECOMMENDED BOOKS

Botanical Medicine for Women's Health by Aviva Romm

RECOMMENDED WEBSITES

Aviva Romm, MD
www.avivaromm.com -

Blessing God's Way
www.blessinggodsway.com

The North American Menopause Society
www.menopause.com

SONGS OF CELEBRATION

Please feel free to copy and distribute the following at your Celebration Gathering to lift your voices together in praise and honor to our King of Kings.

I Surrender All

Judson W. Van DeVenter

Winfield S. Weeden

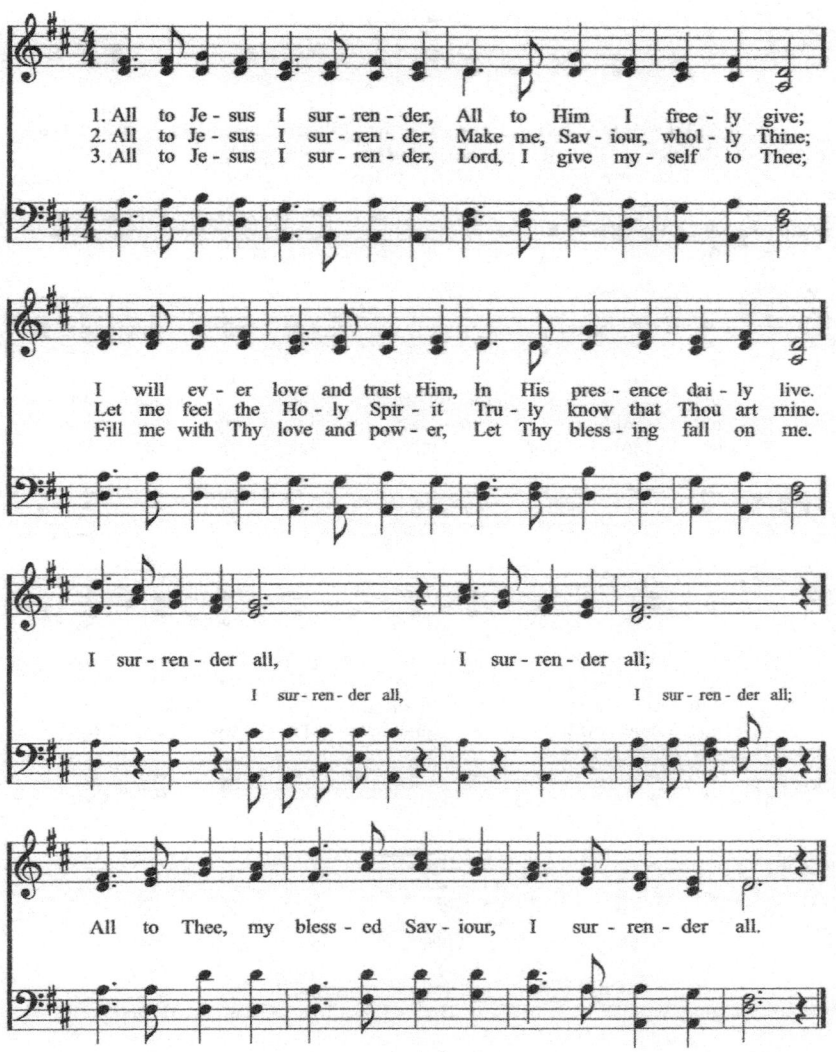

1. All to Je - sus I sur - ren - der, All to Him I free - ly give;
2. All to Je - sus I sur - ren - der, Make me, Sav - iour, whol - ly Thine;
3. All to Je - sus I sur - ren - der, Lord, I give my - self to Thee;

I will ev - er love and trust Him, In His pres - ence dai - ly live.
Let me feel the Ho - ly Spir - it Tru - ly know that Thou art mine.
Fill me with Thy love and pow - er, Let Thy bless - ing fall on me.

I sur - ren - der all, I sur - ren - der all;

I sur - ren - der all, I sur - ren - der all;

All to Thee, my bless - ed Sav - iour, I sur - ren - der all.

Take My Life, and Let It Be

Frances R. Havergal, 1874   Henri A. Cesar Malan, 1827

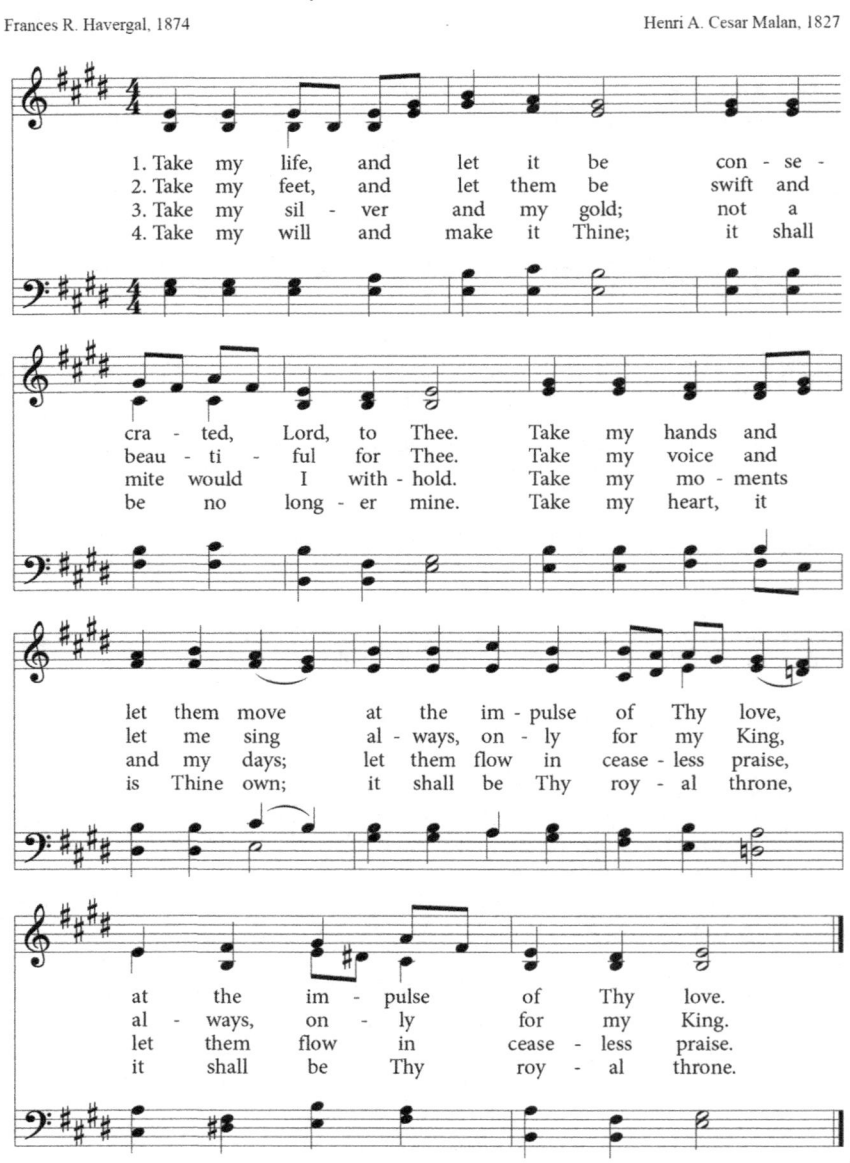

1. Take my life, and let it be con - se -
2. Take my feet, and let them be swift and
3. Take my sil - ver and my gold; not a
4. Take my will and make it Thine; it shall

cra - ted, Lord, to Thee. Take my hands and
beau - ti - ful for Thee. Take my voice and
mite would I with - hold. Take my mo - ments
be no long - er mine. Take my heart, it

let them move at the im - pulse of Thy love,
let me sing al - ways, on - ly for my King,
and my days; let them flow in cease - less praise,
is Thine own; it shall be Thy roy - al throne,

at the im - pulse of Thy love.
al - ways, on - ly for my King.
let them flow in cease - less praise.
it shall be Thy roy - al throne.

To God Be the Glory

Frances Jane (Fanny) Crosby, 1875

William Howard Doane

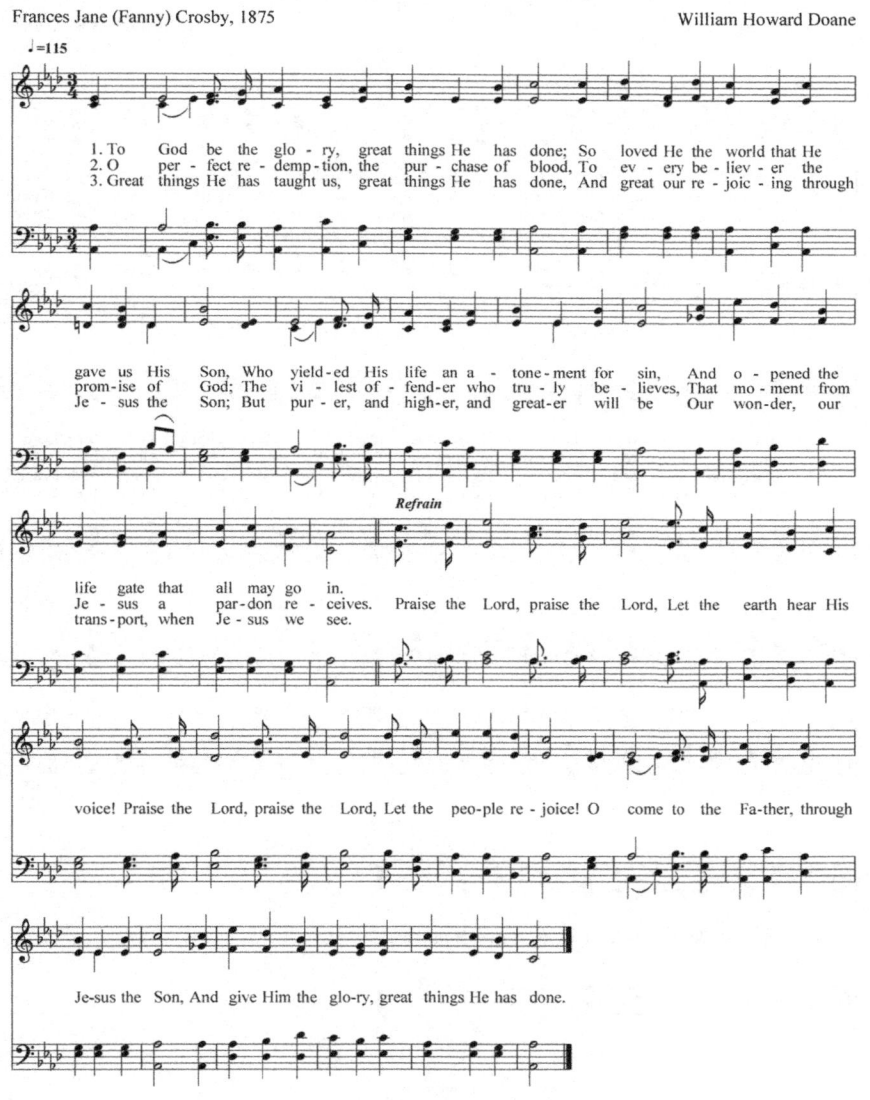

1. To God be the glo - ry, great things He has done; So loved He the world that He gave us His Son, Who yield-ed His life an a - tone-ment for sin, And o - pened the life gate that all may go in.

2. O per - fect re - demp - tion, the pur - chase of blood, To ev - ery be - liev - er the prom-ise of God; The vi - lest of - fend-er who tru - ly be - lieves, That mo - ment from Je - sus a par - don re - ceives.

3. Great things He has taught us, great things He has done, And great our re - joic - ing through Je - sus the Son; But pur - er, and high-er, and great-er will be Our won-der, our trans-port, when Je - sus we see.

Refrain

Praise the Lord, praise the Lord, Let the earth hear His voice! Praise the Lord, praise the Lord, Let the peo-ple re - joice! O come to the Fa-ther, through Je-sus the Son, And give Him the glo-ry, great things He has done.

'Tis So Sweet to Trust in Jesus

Louisa M. R. Stead, 1882

William James Kirkpatrick

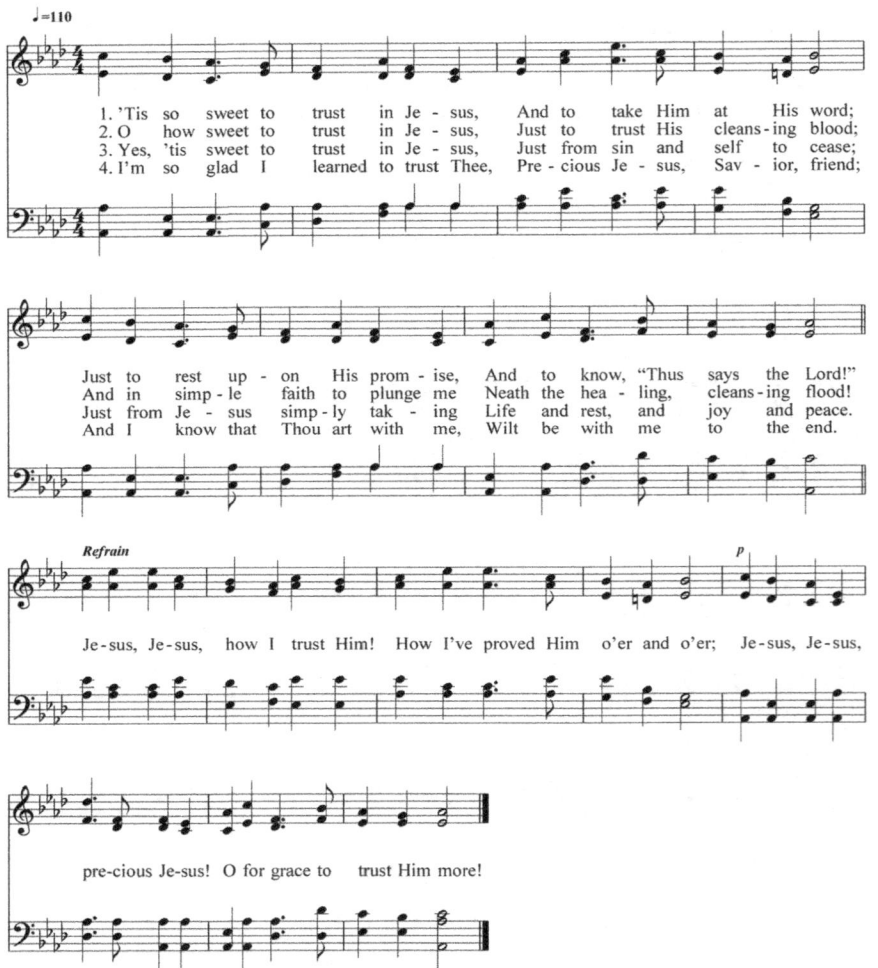

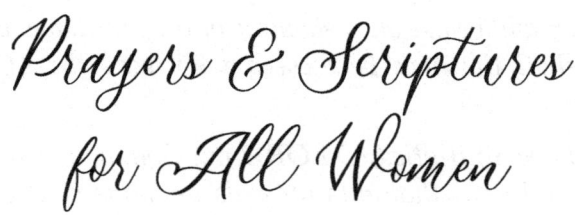

Blessings from God

Prayer

LORD God, our heavenly Father, please help me to be grateful for Your forever loving care towards your children. I thank You for this gift and blessing and rejoice in it. Please help me to be grateful for this design and process, bringing me ever closer to You, my LORD and Savior. Bless Your Holy name for this precious gift. I pray Your blessing throughout this phase in my life, helping me to be a shining light to those around me. Let Your light shine, O God, to those who see me. In Jesus' name, Amen!

Scriptures

"He will bless those who fear the LORD, both the small and the great." Psalm 115:13

"And Mary said, `My soul magnifies the LORD, and my spirit rejoices in God my Savior.'" Luke 1:46-47

"Her children rise up her up and call her blessed; her husband also, and he praises her." Proverbs 31:28

"Blessed is everyone who fears the LORD, who walks in His ways! You shall eat the fruit of the labor of your hands; you shall be blessed, and it shall be well with you. Your wife will be like a fruitful vine within your house; your

children will be like olive shoots around your table. Behold, thus shall the man be blessed who fears the LORD." Psalm 128:1-4

"You have multiplied, O LORD my God, your wondrous deeds and your thoughts towards us; none can compare with you! I will proclaim and tell of them, yet they are more than can be told." Psalm 40:5

"So God created man in His own image, in the image of God He created him; male and female He created them. And God blessed them." Genesis 1:27-28

"Blessed be the God and Father of our Lord Jesus Christ, who has blessed us in Christ with every spiritual blessing in the heavenly places." Ephesians 1:3

Praising God

Prayer

I praise Your Holy Name, Almighty Father. I praise the work You have begun and will complete through Your Son, Jesus Christ. I lift up my hands to You, Who sits on the throne. I want to praise You in the morning and at noon and at night. May the Holy Spirit teach me to praise and worship You for Your continual blessings to my family and me. In Jesus' name, Amen!

Scriptures

"Bless the LORD, O my soul, and all that is within me, bless His holy name! Bless the LORD, O my soul, and forget not all His benefits, who forgives all your iniquity, who heals all your diseases, who redeems your life from the pit, who crowns you with steadfast love and mercy." Psalm 103:1-4

"*Not to us, O LORD, not to us, but to your name give glory, for the sake of your steadfast love and your faithfulness!*" Psalm 115:1

"*It is good to give thanks to the LORD, to sing praises to your name, O Most High; to declare your steadfast love in the morning, and your faithfulness by night, to the music of the lute and the harp, to the melody of the lyre. For you, O LORD, have made me glad by your work; at the works of your hands I sing for joy.*" Psalm 92:1-4

"*Declare His glory among the nations, His marvelous works among all the peoples!*" Psalm 96:3

"*I will bless the LORD at all times; His praise shall continually be in my mouth.*" Psalm 34:1

God's Blessed Design

Prayer

God, You created all things. Your design is perfect in all things. If I focus on Your wonderful works, it will help me to be truly thankful for this design and work in me and around me. You have formed our cycles and bodies; they are wonderfully made, praise be to You. Please help me to acknowledge Your design to those around me. You made heaven and earth and all that is in it; glory be to You, Who sits on high. I pray that You keep this vision before me each and every day, in Jesus' name, Amen!

Scriptures

"*Thus says the LORD, your Redeemer, who formed you from the womb: I am the LORD, who made all things, who alone stretched out the heavens, who spread out the earth by myself.*" Isaiah 44:24,

"For you formed my inward parts; you knitted me together in my mother's womb. I praise you, for I am fearfully and wonderfully made. Wonderful are your works; my soul knows it very well. My frame was not hidden from you, when I was being made in secret, intricately woven in the depths of the earth. Your eyes saw my unformed substance; in your book were written, every one of them, the days that were formed for me, when as yet there was none of them." Psalm 139:13-16

"Before I formed you in the womb, I knew you, and before you were born, I consecrated you; I appointed you a prophet to the nations." Jeremiah 1:5

"He blesses your children within you." Psalm 147:13

"Your hands have fashioned and made me." Job 10:8 96

"For I know the plans that I have for you, declares the LORD, plans for welfare and not for evil, to give you a future and a hope." Jeremiah 29:11

"Your hands have made me and fashioned me; give me understanding, that I may learn your commandments." Psalm 119:73

Peace Within

Prayer

O LORD, my God, in our cycles and different phases of womanhood, we tend to have more anxieties and worries due to the hormones taking off to very high levels at times. I do not want to use this as an excuse to sin. I need to address them, confess them, and trust in You, LORD, that Your grace is sufficient for the season You have me in. Speak to my heart, I pray, to alleviate some of these anxieties, so that I may hold steadfastly to Your timing, joy, and light. Be my strength and my guide, and help me to be ever grateful for the season You have me in. Thank You, Holy Spirit, for Your wisdom and knowledge. In Jesus' name, Amen.

Scriptures

"Be still, and know that I am God." Psalm 46:10

"Do not be anxious about anything, but in everything by prayer and supplication with thanksgiving, let your requests be made known to God. And the peace of God, which surpasses all understanding, will guard your hearts and your minds in Christ Jesus." Philippians 4:6-7

"And do not seek what you are to eat and what you are to drink, nor be worried. For all the nations of the world seek after these things, and your Father knows that you need them. Instead, seek His kingdom, and these things will be added to you." Luke 12:29-31

"Come to me, all who labor and are heavy laden, and I will give you rest. Take my yoke upon you, and learn from me, for I am gentle and lowly in heart, and you will find rest for your souls. For my yoke is easy, and my burden is light." Matthew 11:28-30

Hope & Courage

Prayer

My hope is in You, LORD; my strength is in You, LORD, my life is in You, LORD. It's in You; it's in You. I know that You are sufficient for me. Holy Spirit, fill me with hope for today and the future. I pray for courage to face *each new day as it comes, with the trials and issues that are before me. Let me remember to always give You glory, honor, and praise forevermore! In Jesus' name, Amen!*

Scriptures

"Have I not commanded you? Be strong and courageous. Do not be frightened, and do not be dismayed, for the LORD your God is with you wherever you go." Joshua 1:9

"Hear my cry, O God, listen to my prayer; from the end of the earth I call to You, when my heart is faint. Lead me to the rock that is higher than I." Psalm 61:1-2

"Have you not known? Have you not heard? The LORD is the everlasting God, the Creator of the ends of the earth. He does not faint or grow weary; His understanding is unsearchable. He gives power to the faint, and to him who has no might He increases strength. Even youths shall faint and be weary, and the young men shall fall exhausted, but they who wait for the LORD shall renew their strength; they shall mount up with wings like eagles; they shall run and not be weary, they shall walk and not faint." Isaiah 40:28-31

"The steadfast love of the LORD never ceases; His mercies never come to an end; they are new every morning; great is your faithfulness. The LORD is my portion, says my soul, therefore I will hope in Him." Lamentations 3:22-24

"But He said to me, `My grace is sufficient for you, for my power is made perfect in weakness.'" 2 Corinthians 12:9

"Blessed be the God and Father of our Lord Jesus Christ,

the Father of mercies and God of all comfort, who comforts us in all our affliction..." 2 Corinthians 1:3-4

"I can do all things through Him who strengthens me." Philippians 4:13

"Be strong, and let your heart take courage, all you who wait for the LORD!" Psalm 31:24

"Not that we are sufficient in ourselves to claim anything as coming from us, but our sufficiency is from God." 2 Corinthians 3:5

"Do not be anxious about anything, but in everything by prayer and supplication with thanksgiving, let your requests be made known to God. And the peace of God, which surpasses all understanding, will guard your hearts and your minds in Christ Jesus." Philippians 4:6-7

Never-Ending Faith

Prayer

Heavenly Father, please give me faith. Holy Spirit, fill me with peace, patience, and a positive attitude for all the stages of my life. Your timing is not my timing; grant me the wisdom to really understand that concept. Thank You, LORD God, for Your never-ending watch over me and this phase of womanhood. Give me the grace to do and be what You have called me to be. Your will be done, and not mine own! In Jesus' name, Amen!

Scriptures

"And Jesus answered them, "Have faith in God. Truly, I say to you, whoever says to this mountain, `Be taken up and thrown into the sea,' and does not doubt in his heart, but believes that what He says will come to pass, it will be *done for him. Therefore I tell you, whatever you ask in prayer, believe that you have received it, and it will be yours."* Mark 11:22-24

"Now faith is the assurance of things hoped for, the conviction of things not seen." Hebrews 11:1 "Let us run with endurance the race that is set before us, looking to Jesus, the founder and protector of our faith." Hebrews 12:1-2

"Every good gift and every perfect gift is from above, coming down from the Father of lights, with whom there is no variation or shadow due to change." James 1:17

"And without faith it is impossible to please Him, for whoever would draw near to God must believe that He exists and that He rewards those who seek Him." Hebrews 11:6

Encouragement & Inspiration

Prayer

Your word is encouragement and inspiration to me, LORD. Give me the strength to read your word daily so that it will guide me, by the power of your Holy Spirit. Thank you, Jesus, for being my ultimate encouragement for the work set before me. I love your word and pray the Holy Spirit hides it in my heart to draw upon in time of need. Grant me the inspiration that only you can give your servant. Thank you for this. In Jesus' name, Amen!

Scriptures

"But you, take courage! Do not let your hands be weak, for your work shall be rewarded." 2 Chronicles 15:7

"Wait for the LORD; be strong, and let your heart take

courage; wait for the LORD!" Psalm 27:14

"And we know for those who love God all things work together for good, for those who are the called according to His purpose." Romans 8:28

"I lift up my eyes to the hills. From where does my help come? My help comes from the LORD, Who made heaven and earth." Psalm 121:1-2

"For everything there is a season, a time for every matter under heaven." Ecclesiastes 3:1

"He has made everything beautiful in its time." Ecclesiastes 3:11

"When a woman is giving birth, she has sorrow because her hour has come, but when she has delivered the baby, she no longer remembers the anguish, for joy that a human being has been born into the world. So also you have sorrow now, but I will see you again, and your hearts will rejoice, and no one will take your joy from you." John 16:21-22

"Now to Him who is able to do far more abundantly than all that we ask or think, according to the power at work within us, to Him be glory in the church and in Christ Jesus throughout all generations, forever and ever. Amen." Ephesians 3:20

XII
Final Thoughts

To conclude a book is probably the most daunting aspect of writing. In its completion, it contains finality, hope, desire, and heart. My prayer is that the LORD uses it for His good pleasure. May it bring glory to His name and design for us as women.

My thoughts on ending this guide immediately go to the desire to see women educated on their cycles, their phases of womanhood, and to offer resources to actually implement that education. We need tools to help us stay on the narrow path of life in Christ. We need community. We need to be inspired to carry on with peace, joy, and, most of all, love.

When I was 46, I found out I had cancer—Non-Hodgkin's Lymphoma—and started chemotherapy treatments to beat it. I have been in remission with the knowledge that cancer could come back if the LORD saw fit for that to enter my life as a wife, mother, and midwife again. Being able to put these thoughts on paper and give light to the passion I have in my heart to see women serving women reaches it's culmination through the completion of this book. My heart is to serve Him. I do that by trying to be the best daughter of the King that I can be with what I have. Let's start to celebrate, educate, and support women through their cycles of womanhood, all the while declaring God as the designer of such intricate human beings!

My prayer is that the LORD uses every ounce of this book to bless someone. It is all for Him!

> *"The LORD bless you and keep you; the LORD make His face to shine upon you and be gracious to you; the LORD lift up His countenance upon you and give you peace."* Numbers 6:24-26

About the Author

Doran's love and passion is helping women see that all phases and cycles of womanhood are blessings to us, God's way. She has created resources and tools to help women embrace how our Creator has fearfully & wonderfully made their bodies. She is a Certified Professional Midwife serving women and their families through maternity, birth, and postpartum. She also is the author of a curriculum for girls titled Maidens by His Design. She is a speaker and has been to several international locations where she has used her gifts and passion for holistic women's health. She is also a Shepherd for the Northeast Region for Holy Yoga Instructors. Her yoga training includes: Trauma, Pre/Post Natal, and Yin. She holds a Masters in her yoga certifications.

BLESSINGS GOD'S WAY ministry for women is a universal, international, non-denominational organization with the ultimate goal of to implementing resources on maidenhood, maternity, and menopause within churches, communities, and other organizations that see the importance of proclaiming God as the Creator of women's life cycles.

Our vision is that we desire to glorify God by honoring Him as Creator of the female body and to rejoice in His design for women in all seasons of life. Our mission is to educate, edify, and celebrate God's special plan for women through maidenhood, maternity, and menopause.

Made in the USA
Middletown, DE
20 November 2025

20862219R00070